Praise for *Your Skin, Younger*

"The authors of *Your Skin, Younger* have synthesized hundreds of scientific studies into a clear and concise guide that will help to protect the skin and improve overall health. Along the way, the book illuminates the rich history of nutritional wisdom within the dermatology profession. This multidimensional resource will surely provide valuable lifestyle information for both patients and clinicians alike."
—Ron Moy, MD, President-Elect, American Academy of Dermatology; Past President of the American Society for Dermatology Surgery

"*Your Skin, Younger* brilliantly combines cutting-edge nutrition research with the latest discoveries in the field of dermatology. In addition to being a uniquely informative, practical guide to enjoying more beautiful skin, this landmark book also contains extremely important information that will benefit your overall health and quality of life."
—Susan Biali, MD, Wellness Expert and Author, *Live a Life You Love! 7 Steps to a Healthier, Happier, More Passionate You*

"It is a pleasure to read the compelling historical documentation of the evidence and underlying science behind various supplements and lifestyle changes recommended to keep skin healthy and youthful. This book will be extremely helpful for anyone seeking knowledge and a greater understanding of useful modalities."
—Alan M. Dattner, MD, Founder of HolisticDermatology.com and Editorial Advisor to *Natural Solutions* Magazine

"*Your Skin, Younger* is a delightful read, full of great insight about what's important, and what's not, for the health of your skin. At a time when there is so much misinformation about diet, sun blocks, and cosmeceuticals, these authors have given us reliable facts and figures, nicely presented, and with a phenomenal bibliography. This text will be of significant interest to physicians and the public alike. Congratulations to the authors on

pulling all this useful material together in such an academic, honest, and informative manner."
—Christopher Zachary, MD, Professor and Chair, Department of Dermatology, University of California, Irvine

"This is a wonderful book filled with scientific information and hands-on practical tools to help anyone keep their skin younger and healthier. The best part is that while you are helping your skin, you will end up improving the health of your body and mind."
—Eva M. Selhub, MD, Harvard Medical School, Author, *The Love Response*

"Doctors: Don't be fooled by the delightfully engaging and clear style of this book! *Your Skin, Younger* is a compelling scholarly analysis of the anti-aging effects of diet and lifestyle. Readers: Do not be fooled by the more than 450 scientific references! Logan, Rubin, and Levy charmingly regale you with stories that show you exactly how and why to take care of your skin."
—Valori Treloar, MD, CNS, Founder of Boston's Integrative Dermatology Center and Coauthor, *The Clear Skin Diet*

"The authors have succeeded in cross-linking knowledge from several areas of expertise, making a strong thesis stronger—they have strengthened the public case against the purveyors of sweet poison. Insightful, provocative, science for every man—and every woman."
—F. William Danby, MD, Assistant Professor, Dermatology, Dartmouth Medical School

"The authors of *Your Skin, Younger* are to be applauded for writing this concise, interesting, and informative book. They have carefully reviewed complex disciplines into a readable, understandable, practical, and much more importantly, an 'actionable' set of recommendations for the lay public to promote skin health. Following their recommendations will lead to improved general health, which will be reflected in improved well-being and the desired youthful appearance."
—Anthony A. Gaspari, MD, Professor and Chairman, Department of Dermatology, University of Maryland, School of Medicine

Your Skin, Younger

NEW SCIENCE SECRETS TO NATURALLY YOUNGER SKIN

ALAN C. LOGAN, ND
MARK G. RUBIN, MD
PHILLIP M. LEVY, MD

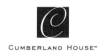

CUMBERLAND HOUSE™

Published by Cumberland House, an imprint of Sourcebooks, Inc.
P.O. Box 4410, Naperville, Illinois 60567-4410
(630) 961-3900
Fax: (630) 961-2168
www.sourcebooks.com

Library of Congress Cataloging-in-Publication Data
Logan, Alan C.
  Your skin, younger : new science secrets to naturally younger skin / Alan C. Logan, Mark G. Rubin, Phillip M. Levy.
     p. cm.
  Includes index.
  1. Skin—Aging. 2. Skin—Care and hygiene. 3. Aging—Nutritional aspects. I. Rubin, Mark G. II. Levy, Phillip M. III. Title.

QP88.5.L64 2009
612.7'9—dc22

2009024573

Printed and bound in the United States of America.
BG 10 9 8 7 6 5 4 3 2 1

This book is dedicated to the Founding Fathers of nutritional dermatology:

John H. Stokes, MD (1885–1961), author of the *Fundamentals of Medical Dermatology*, 1942

Erich Urbach, MD (1893–1946), author of *Skin Diseases, Nutrition, and Metabolism*, 1946

Acknowledgments

ALL AUTHORS WOULD LIKE TO THANK Marcia Hartsock, owner of the Medical Art Company and one of North America's foremost certified medical illustrators. We would also like to thank two librarians, Eisha Prather of Cornell University and Barbara Mathieu of Washington University, St. Louis, who went above and beyond the call of duty in helping us to secure difficult-to-find journal or newspaper archives.

The authors are also extremely grateful for the guidance and inspiration of dermatologist Dr. Alan M. Dattner. For the last thirty years, Dr. Dattner has been a leading voice and proponent of a holistic and integrative approach in dermatology. Founder of HolisticDermatology.com, Dr. Dattner has been writing, researching, and speaking on the values of nutritional medicine for skin care long before it was in vogue to do so.

In addition, we are extremely grateful for the support of Sourcebooks, and, in particular, Editor Sara Kase who worked tirelessly to sculpt this book.

CONTENTS

Introduction

HUMAN BEINGS HAVE TAKEN STEPS TO beautify the skin since time immemorial. Some historians have argued that the use of colorful ochre-based medicinal cosmetics may even predate humans, going back 1.5 million years to *Homo erectus*. Whoever first discovered medicinal cosmetics is the unsung hominid that started it all—a 200-billion-dollar global empire designed to beautify, protect, and heal.

Today such efforts are paired with a great deal of sophistication, pharmaceutical-driven science, technological advances, and marketing embellishment. A dizzying array of almost ten thousand chemicals (the bulk of them synthetic) appear in skin-care products. Confusion abounds, and, in many ways, we have lost touch with the roots of beauty, turning our backs on the true medicinal aspects of cosmetic intervention and the wisdom of our elders.

The fundamental nutritional aspects of internally and externally promoting youthful, glowing skin have been known for decades. Yet, with the advent of pharmaceuticals and cutting-edge technological advances in the 1950s and 1960s, these important considerations were relegated to the fringes of dermatological sciences. But nutritional cosmetic research is no longer entirely on the sidelines. In this book, we will discuss some of the most exciting research studies in recent years, investigations that are paving the way for new developments in nutritional dermatology.

Right from the start, we will dismantle the myth that a wrinkle is just a wrinkle, a benign part of the aging process that we should just let happen. Visible signs of aging are far from benign; they are legitimate markers of the internal condition of the human body. We will also dismantle the myth that visible signs of aging are simply a matter of sun and genetics. You don't have to look old for your age.

Despite all the advances of cosmetic dermatology, and despite our ability to erase a significant portion of these external markers of aging, we simply cannot ignore the need for a deeper aspect of care—one that improves the skin while slowing the actual aging process, both inside and out. The most powerful aspect of medicine is prevention, and we will discuss in great detail the many ways in which the skin's aging process can be slowed, as well as the unhealthy ways in which it is accelerated.

Emerging studies show that certain dietary items protect against the visible signs of aging, but the reality of the North American diet often causes us to shun protective agents found in foods and beverages. Research shows that we live in denial about our own dietary habits, assuming that we generally eat healthy, while it is "everybody else" that needs a change. We hope the candid discussions in this book about diet and the visible signs of aging will encourage you to make a change, to make the foods and drinks that protect against skin aging the rule, rather than the exception, and to minimize your intake of foods that attack the long-term health of the skin layers.

The problem is not just the foods we eat—but also how we prepare them. Often articles in magazines and on websites are devoted to healthy skin foods, yet there is no discussion about how food preparation impacts the health of the skin and its aging process. We will introduce you to an entirely new concept that is ignored by beauty experts, even those who claim to be nutrition experts: Advanced Glycation End-products, or aptly named AGEs, in foods that are cooked on high heat in the absence of moisture. These food-based AGEs cause inflammation and oxidative stress and attack your collagen.

With the recipes in this book provided by Tokyo native Yoshiko Sato, we will help you end this vicious AGE nutritional cycle by taking a leaf out of Japanese food preparation. Until now, beauty experts have focused primarily on the fact that too much dietary sugar could cause collagen-damaging glycation in the skin. As you will see, turning off the oven, using a steamer, and poaching, boiling, simmering, or stewing your foods can go a long way in the effort to maintain a youthful and glowing appearance. In the coming years, we expect AGEs in food to be considered as important as the food's fat or sugar content.

The intestinal tract is an organ that can make or break youthful skin. For more than a century, researchers have made connections among healthy gut bacteria, healthy skin, and the aging process itself. It may seem implausible that your gut could have anything other than a minimal impact on the condition of the skin. Yet in many ways, so-called friendly intestinal-tract bacteria can positively influence skin health and minimize chemicals that promote the development of visible signs of aging. We will discuss these complex pathways in straightforward and understandable terms. By the time you are finished with the gut-skin chapter, you will agree that yogurt, fermented foods, and other sources of good bacteria are the skin's best friend.

Any book that attempts to discuss nutritional skin care—or nutritional aspects of any disease, for that matter—in the absence of stress and lifestyle considerations is an incomplete work. Nutrition simply cannot be isolated from stress, and vice versa. In addition, chronic stress and sleep problems undoubtedly contribute to the visible signs of aging. Chronic stress also contributes to our eating habits: we aren't reaching for broccoli and kale when stress looms big. No, we reach for foods cooked with high AGE techniques that contribute to the skin's aging processes. In this book, we will uncover specific pathways by which stress and stress-induced dietary alterations can push the skin-aging process. We also discuss in detail mind-body medical interventions that can be used to combat the cycle of stress-induced aging. Nutrition can improve mental outlook and provide a layer of insulation against the modern stress load.

Finally, we will take you on a journey through the world of dietary supplements and natural, topical nutrients that can feed the skin.

Attempting to feed the skin with supplements or topicals, or both, requires entering a world filled with endless choices and marketing hype. We aim to take away some of the confusion and pare down the need to take bags of supplements. We will also provide guidance on the fast-paced research surrounding the natural cosmetics industry.

For years, consumers have been like marionettes dancing to the tune of the string-holding marketers within the colossal cosmetics industry. Lured by the promise of so-called youth ingredients and other such trademarked nonsense, consumers have been kept in the dark about the safety, true efficacy, and environmental impact of the chemicals applied to the skin. We will teach you to become a wise consumer, one who questions everything related to feeding the skin. Our guidance is based on the synthesis of thousands of scientific publications and decades of combined clinical experience.

While the marketing efforts of some companies still seem to lie ahead of their research and development accomplishments, a growing number of nutrients have been the subject of solid, published research. The research on some natural ingredients is beginning to validate the historical aspects of ingredient choices for skin care. There is much to be excited about, such as topical cosmetics that work, are sustainable and environmentally friendly, and most importantly, are safe for consumers.

At times, this type of material can become deep and complex, but in this book, the messages will remain straightforward, readable, and comprehensive in need-to-know information. We will not leave anything out, and the in-depth discussions let you know this is not just another pop-health book. The last thing the world needs is another superficial book telling readers to eat healthy without allowing them to understand how and why this is so important. An in-depth analysis with historical perspective provides a true understanding of the mechanisms by which diet, food preparation, and lifestyle can interact in the promotion (or destruction) of youthful skin.

These are indeed exciting times when it comes to the prevention of skin aging. The good news is that more and more young and middle-aged people are refusing to stand idly by and watch visible signs of aging unfold without a fight. In *Your Skin, Younger*, our first priority is to underscore that nutrition and lifestyle matter. For young adults, eating healthy, nutritious foods and keeping stress in check is much easier if the endgame is the maintenance of youthful skin. Follow the practices and interventions we advocate in this book, and ultimately not only will you slow visible signs of aging and improve the condition of the skin, but you will also be in a much better position to navigate the overall aging process, remain engaged in life, and maintain a high quality of life, which researchers call successful aging.

The combined authorship of two dermatologists and a naturopathic physician is a rare one. Our training and backgrounds differ, yet they converge in our desire to help our patients in all ways possible. Two of us are dermatologists specializing in cosmetic dermatology who have spent countless hours on advanced training in the unique aspects of pharmaceutical and technological anti-aging interventions for the skin. Added to that is the expertise of a licensed naturopathic physician trained in natural methods to maintain youthful skin.

Nutrition is the cornerstone of naturopathic medicine. Licensure requires more than 220 hours of classroom nutritional training and countless hours of nutritional counseling in a required clinical setting. Perhaps most importantly, licensure as a naturopathic physician (in those states and provinces that are regulated) requires the passage of individual board exams in which 100 percent of the questions are devoted specifically to biochemical and clinical nutrition. Therefore, just as any book devoted to anti-aging skin care should involve the guidance of seasoned cosmetic dermatologists, such books delving into the topics of nutrition, botanicals, and mind-body medicine should involve the guidance of a credentialed naturopath.

The result is a complete, natural action plan for the maintenance of youthful skin. Our discussions and the interventions we advocate are not a substitute for appropriate dermatological care and evaluation. Used with the advice of your dermatologist, however, our recommendations are key pieces of the puzzle of true holistic care. We hope this book serves as a template for shared discussion and decision-making in the long-term care of your skin and what lies beneath.

Yours in Health!

Alan C. Logan, ND   Mark G. Rubin, MD   Phillip M. Levy, MD

1

Inside Out:
The Renewed Science of Dermatology

SUN EXPOSURE IS A MAJOR CONTRIBUTOR to the visible signs of aging. That's common knowledge. Outside of this fact, however, most adults—even doctors—write off youthful-looking skin as a simple matter of genetics. The assumption is that fine lines, wrinkles, dullness, furrows, sagging, uneven tone, roughness, and scaling are a matter of the cards that have been dealt from the genetic deck. Many people think that these visible signs of skin aging should be accepted as a foregone conclusion, that we should just sit idly by and watch them unfold in the mirror as a "normal" part of the aging process. But that's not true.

Nutrition, stressors, mental outlook, lifestyle habits, and other environmental factors all play a role in the visible signs of aging. Genetics are far from the whole story, and much can be done from a nutritional standpoint, both internally and topically, to combat and prevent the aging processes in human skin. Visible signs of aging should not be dismissed as benign. In addition to the tremendous psychological fallout, a growing body of science demonstrates that facial wrinkles are a reliable surrogate marker of internal health.

Using nutrition and lifestyle approaches, we will help you complement the outstanding technological advances used in dermatology clinics and promote health from the inside out. Cutting-edge techniques of cosmetic dermatology provide an incredible service to patients who want to undo the hands of time. The satisfaction rating of those who seek dermatological care for nonsurgical cosmetic medicine is extremely high. The advances in technology and sophistication of treatments have translated into meaningful visual results, which in turn translate into improved self-esteem and quality of life.

Much has been written on advances in laser techniques, microdermabrasion, botox injections, and injectable fillers, to name a few. Countless books and articles describe the anti-aging advantages of modern dermatological care. Here we will take a different approach, one that takes us back to the future in dermatology. Some sixty or seventy years ago, great emphasis was placed on the effect of nutrition and lifestyle on the health and appearance of skin. There was an inside-out approach to healthy skin.

As the scientific sophistication of dermatology shifted into high gear in the 1960s, many of the older teachings were, as one dermatologist put it, "thrown into the dustbin of history." The focus shifted almost exclusively to synthetic topical preparations and light-based technology. Nutrition had no place in this new paradigm and was quickly relegated to the stuff of home economics class. Yet today, research has validated many of the teachings of our dermatology elders, and nutrition and lifestyle are back in scientific vogue. In addition to radiant, glowing skin with diminished signs of aging, many collateral health benefits come with consideration of diet and stress management. As you work your way through these chapters, you will be armed with the knowledge to boldly resist the opposing forces of skin aging.

Holding Us Together

Everything in your body is contained, or held in, by a tremendous organ with great sophistication, durability, and resiliency—your skin. Many of us take the skin for granted. When we think of a human organ, we tend to think of the brain, heart, kidneys, or lungs. Rarely do we sit back and appreciate our skin as a living, breathing, and dynamic organ. It is our largest organ: spread out, it covers some 20 square feet, and it makes up one-sixth of average body weight. But skin just doesn't get the respect it deserves.

Over the course of a lifetime, our skin will do so much for us, not the least of which is its service as the great defender against the assaults of the outside world. It is also involved in fluid and temperature control, immune system surveillance, vitamin D formation, and the transfer of sensory information. It is our organ of emotional expression; facial skin allows the visual display of all our deepest emotions. You can think of your skin as a brave soldier on the front lines, protecting you from all conceivable physical, chemical, and environmental assaults.

How do we repay this brave soldier for its acts of valor? Do we care for the skin and provide it with all of the raw materials for optimal functioning? What type of rations and nourishment do we provide? What type of rest from stress is provided? Do we place the skin in harm's way more often than need be? Do we damage the skin with dangerous synthetic chemicals purported to help skin structure and function? The answers to all of these questions will determine the true "age" of your skin, a numerical value quite distinct from your chronological age.

High-quality human nutrition provides all the raw materials necessary for both structure and functioning of the skin, and a steady stream of optimal nutrients go a long way in supporting healthy skin over the course of a lifetime. Nutrient deficiencies, on the other hand, can compromise skin health, and dietary excesses in the form of sugar and harmful fast food can directly damage skin structure and function.

Anatomy

Before considering aging skin's structural and physiological changes and how to limit the aging process, we must first look at the components of normal skin.

EPIDERMIS: THE OUTER LAYER

The outer layer of the skin, the part we actually see, is the epidermis. Although very thin, usually only half a millimeter, depending on location, the epidermis contains the important components on the next page. Renewing the epidermis takes about four weeks in normal skin. As we age, this turnaround time increases by as much as 50 percent, while the demand for nutrients becomes even more important.

- *Stratum Corneum:* Set up like bricks and mortar, this layer within the epidermis is critical for moist, well-hydrated skin. The stratum corneum is made up of keratin (bricks) and intercellular lipid complex (mortar).
- *Ceramides:* These are fat- (or lipid-) based chemicals within the stratum corneum. Some cosmetics mimic these ceramides, since they maintain the skin barrier.
- *Keratin:* This tough protein provides flexibility, chemical resistance, and protection. It is made up of nutrients such as amino acids, carbohydrates, and fatty acids.
- *Basal Layer:* Located at the bottom of the epidermis, this layer creates cells that form keratin.
- *Melanocytes:* These cells in the basal layer produce melanin, our skin pigment.
- *Langerhans Cells:* These cells perform immune system surveillance.

DERMIS: THE SCAFFOLDING

Here we have important structural components of the skin—the scaffolding, if you will. This mesh network of connective tissues has a heavy workload in maintaining the appearance of the skin. Problems with any of the principal components of the dermis contribute to visible signs of aging. Problems at all levels spell disaster.

- *Collagen:* A key player in connective tissue, it provides strength.
- *Elastin:* Another key player in connective tissue, providing turgor, or the ability to stretch and spring back and return to position.
- *Glycosaminoglycans (GAGs):* The Volumizers
  This group of key players provides elasticity and volume. Hyaluronic acid (HA), the major GAG, makes up 70 percent of the total and is a well-known nutrient in cosmetic care. HA acts as a sponge, holding up to one thousand times its own weight in water. Researchers recently discovered that GAGs are not simply structural. They also act as a major antioxidant in the dermis.
- *Fibroblasts:* Dermal cells that manufacture collagen and elastin.

- *Sweat Glands*: These are made up of hair follicles, sebaceous glands that secrete an oily substance called sebum, and immune system channels called lymphatic vessels.

DERMAL-EPIDERMAL JUNCTION: THE BLOOD SOURCE

This is a distinct wave-like band of *rete ridges*, or interlocking projections that spread out and increase the surface area of the epidermis so that it can receive its maximum complement of nutrient- and oxygen-rich blood.

SUBCUTANEOUS TISSUE: THE SHOCK ABSORBER

The bottom layer of the skin, the subcutaneous layer, sits on our muscles, and the muscles on our bones. That is not an insignificant fact with regard to skin appearance because loss of muscle and bone through the aging process can certainly influence skin appearance. The subcutaneous tissue consists mostly of *fat cells*, the main provider of insulation and shock absorption.

Skin Changes Induced by Aging

With the background of normal skin anatomy in place, let's turn our attention to what happens in the skin layers when marked visible signs of aging present themselves. What are the differences when we look at the skin of a young person and compare it to the skin layers associated with fine lines, wrinkles, furrows, sagging, discoloration, and dark circles? Changes characteristic of the aging process shift into high gear when skin is influenced by various factors, ultraviolet sunlight exposure being only one of them.

The sun-induced aging process, called photoaging, and an unchecked biological aging of the skin (supplemented with stress, a poor diet, and smoking) will both give you the same older-looking face. While some differences exist between photoaging and unbridled biologically aged skin, the differences are really a matter of semantics. For example, the epidermis in photoaging may be thicker because it is crusted and malformed. However, it has also been known to thin out in the manner characteristic of biological skin aging. Both photoaging and biological aging affect the skin to create visible aging.

> **Stratum Corneum:** The barrier layer within the epidermis. Set up like a brick-and-mortar wall, its normal structure is essential in keeping the skin well hydrated.

A breakdown in the stratum corneum is characteristic of the skin-aging process and results in greater water loss and dehydration in aged skin. Another big change in aged skin is the flattening of rete ridges—the interlocking finger-like projections between the epidermis and dermis. When the ridges flatten out, surface area is lost and blood flow to the region declines considerably. This is especially bad because the aging process already causes diminished volume of blood delivered by the blood vessels.

The overall decrease in blood flow ultimately translates to a decline in important antioxidant and anti-inflammatory nutrients, and the removal of metabolic waste also declines. Like an appliance company that brings you the new washer and dryer and hauls away the old rusty ones, your blood delivers new nutrients and hauls away the junk. But your blood can only perform this service if it can gain access to the residence, in this case, your skin cells.

Within the aging dermis is a disorganization of collagen fibers, and while overall elastic tissue may increase, its structure is discombobulated. When the scaffolding of any structure starts to become disorganized, it loses stability and things crumble. In the case of aging skin, the propensity to wrinkle and sag is greatly enhanced when the skin's structure becomes disorganized. While most scientific attention regarding aged dermis focuses on collagen and elastin, there is also a noticeable loss of those important GAGs (glycosaminoglycans).

> **Glycosaminoglycans:** These supportive structures within the dermis help keep collagen in place and draw in moisture. The chief GAG, hyaluronate, can hold one thousand times its weight in water. The GAGs provide volume, hydration, and firmness through the aging process.

Loss of bone integrity, muscle mass, and subcutaneous fat all contribute to the appearance of visible signs of aging. All of these structures lie below the epidermis and dermis, so you might not immediately think of them as part of the problem. Yet they add to the picture of aging by taking away the "fullness" and definition of facial structure. Osteoporosis experts have noted that loss of facial bone mass is an underappreciated cause of an older appearance, as compared to adults who maintain healthy bones. Young adults have an even distribution of fat tissue. The aging process enhances the likelihood of "pocket" accumulation of facial fat. Throw in a chaser of gravitational force on these cordoned-off areas of fat, and a droop, sag, and jowl is born.

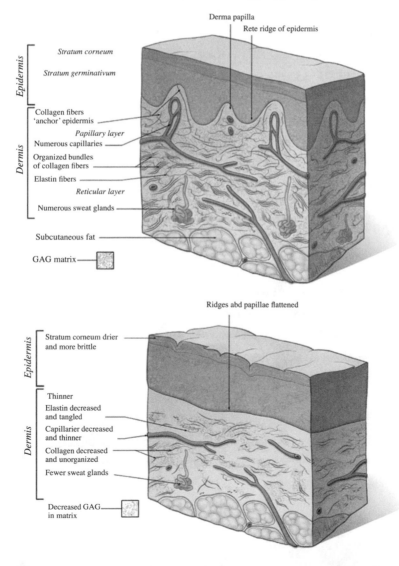

Accelerated Skin Aging

If you want to see the skin-aging process in overdrive, look at the skin under the toxic influences of what is called *extrinsic aging*.

> **Extrinsic Aging:** The skin aging that develops as a result of external factors. The primary culprit of extrinsic aging is, as you probably know, ultraviolet (UV) radiation from sun exposure.

UV RADIATION

UV radiation hits our skin in the form of damaging UVA and UVB rays. Try this mnemonic device to remember the difference—UVA for Aging and UVB for Bad Burn. UVB gives you the redness typical of a sunburn. The SPF, or sun protective factor number, of a sunscreen refers to its ability to block out UVB radiation. Most of the UVB is absorbed and eliminated at the epidermal layer, but not without causing some real problems first. It damages the DNA of the keratin-producing keratinocytes, markedly reducing the production of new DNA for several hours after exposure.

> **Keratin:** A tough protein providing flexibility, chemical resistance, and protection. Made up of nutrients such as amino acids, carbohydrates, and fatty acids.

The DNA damage induced by UVB rays has been associated with an increased risk of various skin cancers.

UVA radiation is the real culprit in accelerating the visible signs of aging. Unlike UVB, which is mostly absorbed and eliminated at the epidermis, UVA passes through the epidermis to the dermis, where it runs amok. Even mild sun exposure, not enough to induce overt sunburn, can cause a massive increase in enzymes called *matrix metalloproteinases* (MMPs).

> **Matrix Metalloproteinases (MMPs):** Enzymes responsible for the breakdown of collagen. Think of them as scissors snipping away at the dermal structures.

Any agent—sun, stress, air pollutants, poor diet, or otherwise—that can energize the enzymes responsible for cutting apart your collagen is not a good thing. To make matters worse, collagen production grinds to a halt and oxidative stress in the dermis is elevated when MMPs start working overtime. The end result is that our collagen becomes fragmented and disoriented.

You can think of normal collagen fiber strands as three ropes neatly wrapped around each other. This is not the case when the strands are subjected to oxidative stress and environmental damage. The collagen fibers become thinned out in certain areas, and partial deterioration is evident. They also start clumping together. The elastin starts to grow thicker. This may seem like a good thing, but more elastin is not necessarily better because it forms clumps and turns into a globular mess.

With repeated exposure come misguided attempts by enzymes to repair the dire situation, and these local patchwork repair efforts only worsen the structure of collagen and elastin. Blood flow diminishes overall, but in certain areas of the skin, blood flow appears to be closer to the surface because the skin has thinned out. This leads to areas of discoloration and a loss of a normal, youthful tone. Interestingly, even skin tone is the first major factor considered, after the absence of wrinkles, when people attempt to determine the chronological age of a third party.

FACIAL ATTRIBUTES IN AGE ESTIMATION

A number of studies have shown that humans constantly size each other up for health and vitality. In this sizing-up process, third-party evaluators of age, health, and vitality consistently use facial attributes as surrogate markers of age, health, and vitality. Here are the top five:

1. Mouth area: wrinkles around the lips
2. Eye area: wrinkles and dark circles
3. Overall skin tone: uneven coloration, presence of brown spots
4. Nasolabial fold: the so-called parentheses sign around the nose and mouth
5. Frown lines: forehead wrinkles

OTHER ENVIRONMENTAL FACTORS

In addition to UV dangers, other damaging environmental factors include but are not limited to smoking, air pollution, ozone exposure, and the electromagnetic frequencies generated by cell phones and smartphones—or as we call them, *crack*berries. We will discuss this in more detail in chapter 2. For now, suffice it to say that any number of environmental factors are at play, and while UV exposure gets all the attention, it is by no means the whole story. For example, the interplay of nutrition and UV exposure has been garnering increased research support.

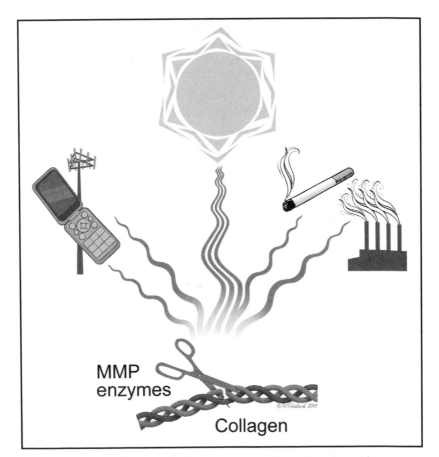

Sun, smoking, stress, pollution, and electromagnetic radiation increase oxidative stress and inflammation in the skin. The result is a potential increase in the activity of MMP enzymes that can cut away at your collagen. Nutrition and lifestyle choices can slow down these runaway enzymes.

It is interesting to note that in the late 1960s, scientific journal articles referred to UV exposure as accounting for almost 100 percent of the nongenetic, external influences on the visible signs of aging. Then, when study after study showed that smoking induces facial wrinkling, the sun's contribution to skin aging dropped to "more than 90" percent. Take into consideration the emerging studies we will discuss next, those related to disease, diet, job strain, mood state, and stress, and the sun's contribution has been estimated at 80 percent and falling fast.

> The first scientist to document marked changes in the dermal skin tissue via sun exposure did so about one hundred years ago. Charles J. White, MD, Harvard's chief of dermatology, published his findings in the *Journal of Cutaneous Disease* (1910). He concluded that states of disease in older adults are associated with marked changes to the elastic tissue. While he connected sun exposure to changes In the elastic fibers of the dermis, he also acknowledged that other environmental factors were at play as well.

"He Looks Old for His Age"

Why are visible signs of aging—fine lines, wrinkles, sagging, roughness and scaling, and overall discoloration—apparent in someone thirty years old and virtually absent in someone fifty-five years old? You may think that the fifty-five-year-old with the youthful, vibrant skin has great genetics and stays out of the sun, which would be the easy answer. But recent advances in the science of aging skin reveal that the exclusivity of wrinkles to genetics and sun may be a bit simplistic. That's not to say that genetics and sun exposure don't matter—they absolutely do. However, other factors are also at play. Scientific advances show that diet and lifestyle exert significant control over genes. The foods we eat, the beverages we drink, and the stressors we experience can all combine to influence what is called *genetic expression*.

> **Genetic Expression:** Environmental factors controlling the degree to which one may experience a genetically mediated medical disease or whether one gets the disease at all.

Environmental factors affecting genetic expression include diet, stress, history of trauma, mental health, and toxic exposures. These factors all interact with genes as we proceed through life. Countless examples in medical literature show how environmental factors influence genetic expression. Twin studies routinely show that, despite genetic predisposition, one twin will often not experience a disease or chronic medical condition, while the other will succumb to it. The influence of lifestyle, diet, stress, and environmental toxins has been documented in all aspects of medicine—from mental health disorders to gastrointestinal disease—and, of course, in dermatological conditions.

Other people use the condition of your skin as a visual cue to assess chronological age, health, and vitality. While this fact may be dismissed as just another example of our youth-obsessed culture and the prevalence of insidious ageism, the reality runs deeper. Evolutionary psychologists have demonstrated time and time again that both sexes are wired to visually assess health and vitality. So when it comes to the visible signs of facial aging, we are fairly good at sizing up overall internal health. Using those visual cues as a surrogate marker for internal health turns out to be quite reliable.

Harry Daniell, MD, an internist working in Redding, California, uncovered an interesting link between internal disease and wrinkles in a study published in the *Annals of Internal Medicine* (1971). For years, he was convinced that smoking caused facial wrinkles in his patients. After a one-year study of more than one thousand community residents, aged thirty to seventy, Daniell did indeed show that smoking greatly increased the risk of wrinkles—even more than sun exposure, according to his results.

Yet one intriguing finding was, at the time, almost inexplicable. Among male smokers over age fifty, those who had the worst wrinkle scores were also those who had a higher prevalence of certain diseases—this when compared to smokers with the same smoking habits and the least wrinkles. Specifically, Daniell found that the smokers who had the least wrinkles were twice as likely *not* to have a history of heart attacks, strokes, or both. Even though these men smoked the same number of cigarettes for the same length of time, and even though they were the same age and gender, those with the greatest wrinkling had double the risk of these potentially fatal events.

Around the same time, aging expert Alex Comfort, PhD, of University College, London, was making a strong argument that microscopic examination of skin tissue could provide an excellent inferential test for overall human aging. Well known for establishing the first battery of clinical tests to estimate the human aging rate, Comfort relied heavily upon skin markers in the process. Specifically he used skin elasticity, collagen contraction, and fibroblast growth as key aspects in making objective measurements of aging. A few years later, dermatological scientist Gary Grove, PhD, found that human volunteers who were perceived to be older looking actually had much slower rates of skin healing. The older-looking volunteers had a marked reduction in the capacity of the outer skin layers to reproduce.

To underscore how visual cues can translate into perception of age and actual human health, researchers from the Gerontology Research Center in Baltimore set up an interesting experiment. They asked medical doctors to guess a person's age based on a quick visual assessment. The doctors had no knowledge of the patient's medical background or personal data; they also had no specialized training in visual-cue assessment. The results of the perception-based age guess, involving more than one thousand adults, were subsequently evaluated alongside known markers of chronic disease risk, including blood tests, neurological testing, and so on.

The results, published in the journal *Social Science and Medicine* (1982), showed that in follow-up, the participants who were rated as looking "older for their age" were much more likely to die at a faster rate from various causes. Indeed, the visual perception of looking older was also associated with results of blood tests and other objective testing known to be markers of risk for chronic disease. In the study, the authors pointed out that wrinkles would obviously have been one of the cues used in visual assessment.

A more specific and recent investigation into facial aging and health was conducted by Kaare Christensen, MD, PhD, and colleagues from the Danish Twin Registry. This was a really neat study; published in the journal *Epidemiology* (2004), it looked at about one hundred sets of older adult twins whose faces had been digitally photographed with neutral expressions. Third-party evaluators, twenty nurses in this case, used the photographs to guess the age of each individual twin. In the years following, the researchers found that, among the twins, the individual twin who had been assessed as older looking was more likely to die from various health-related causes in 73 percent of the cases.

Further analysis of the perceived age of the twins indicated that genetic influence is not even close to the whole story of the visible signs of aging. Actually, genetics were estimated to account for only about half of the end result in facial appearance. If genetics were the whole story, then these older twin pairs should have had identical facial aging. But they didn't. So, the next time you are told that someone has great skin because of his or her genes, tell him or her it isn't so simple.

> **Remember:** Diet, environmental exposures, stressors, and lifestyle habits can influence the genes that influence the condition of your skin.

Martalena Purba, PhD, and colleagues from Monash University in Australia examined wrinkling at skin sites *with only limited sun exposure* to determine if wrinkling might be used as a surrogate marker for overall health status. Close to five hundred older adults were assessed via measures of skin wrinkling, tests of mental well-being, and blood work for a hormone associated with health and vitality called dehydroepiandrosterone (DHEA), a hormone that drops in level during the aging process.

The researchers found that the greater the degree of skin wrinkling, the lower the scores of general health (for conditions such as diabetes, heart disease, and hypertension) and overall functional status. They also found that those with the lowest degree of wrinkling had the highest blood levels of DHEA. Remember, these findings were based on assessments of skin wrinkling at skin sites not usually exposed to significant UV rays!

Other investigative groups have linked facial wrinkling with lung disease, and more recently, facial wrinkles were shown to predict poor kidney function. In the study published in *Nephrology* (2008), Korean researchers found that facial wrinkling was associated with a reduced kidney-filtration rate. This link was independent of age and gender, and once again, the researchers controlled for the potential bias of smoking-associated wrinkles and kidney function. They also eliminated the influence of sun exposure, diabetes, and other wrinkle-inducing confounding factors.

The Korean group showed a major link among reduced kidney filtration, wrinkles, and body-wide oxidative stress. In this case, blood markers of oxidative stress were much higher in those who had facial wrinkles, and the connection was a linear one. Higher levels of oxidative stress markers in the blood were associated with higher risk of overall wrinkles and greater severity and depth of wrinkles. Once again, looking old was linked to internal problems—in this case, a decreased ability to filter out toxins from the human body. (The concept of free-radical damage and increased oxidative stress in wrinkle induction will be taken up in detail in chapter 2.)

In sum, these studies show us that visible signs of aging are a potential mirror of internal health, and should not be dismissed offhand as an issue for celebrities and the vain who succumb to the pressures of our pop culture–driven society. Health and vitality are truly reflected in our skin. The benefits of good-looking skin are many, not the least of which is a potentially extended life with greater quality.

Diet, Workload, and Mental Outlook

Eating bad foods greatly enhances the risk of chronic diseases—diabetes, osteoporosis, and heart disease, as well as neurological and even psychiatric disorders. Chronic stress increases the risk of these same chronic diseases. Likewise, chronic disease significantly increases the risk of mental-health symptoms and chronic stress. Have these diet and stress connections been associated with wrinkles? The answer is yes, positively.

People have talked about the possible connection between diet and wrinkles over the years. Most notably, Manhattan dermatologist Irwin I. Lubowe, MD, was a major proponent of a diet-wrinkle connection in the 1980s. But it wasn't until 2001 that solid and specific diet-wrinkle patterns emerged, highlighted in another study by Dr. Purba and colleagues at Monash University.

The Australian researchers had confirmed a link between health status and wrinkles, but they also wanted to see if wrinkles might be associated with specific dietary patterns. They looked at the diets of close to five hundred older adults and found that the foods we promote to reduce chronic disease, cardiovascular disease, diabetes, and so forth, are the same foods that appear to protect against wrinkles. They didn't prove that these healthy foods stop wrinkles. In the study, published in the *Journal of the American College of Nutrition* (2001), they made what epidemiologists call a correlation or an association.

> **The Diet-Wrinkle Correlation:** Independent of sun and other environmental factors, a consistent diet in healthy foods is associated with significantly fewer wrinkles and visible signs of facial aging.

Specifically, the researchers found that the older adults with the highest intake of items like olive oil, fish and seafood, nuts, legumes, yogurt, tea, whole-grain cereals, deep-green vegetables, and dark fruits and berries had the fewest visible signs of aging. These high-value foods are rich in fiber, antioxidants, and anti-inflammatory nutrients. On the other hand, a greater risk of skin wrinkling was associated with consumption of fatty, processed meats, butter, margarine, dairy fat, saturated fats, white potatoes, sugary beverages (think soda), and sweet, sugary desserts.

The Monash group is not the only set of investigators who have studied diet and wrinkles and documented a connection. Maeve Cosgrove, PhD, and colleagues reported in the *American Journal of Clinical Nutrition* (2007) that too much fat in general, too many carbohydrates, and not enough vitamin C and protein were associated with wrinkles in more than four thousand adults at least forty years old. Dermatologists assessed dryness, wrinkles, and thinning, or atrophy, of the skin. Higher vitamin C intake was associated with protection against wrinkling and dry skin—not shocking when you consider that vitamin C is vital in the formation of collagen. These findings were independent of known wrinkle-inducing elements like sun and smoking.

Further evidence comes from a study by Spanish researchers in 2009; after completing detailed lifestyle questionnaires, 252 women (ages 30–70) were digitally photographed and evaluated for age by fifty-five third-party adults. Among the most significant lifestyle factors associated with a younger appearance: a healthy diet and quality sleep.

COMMON UV MYTHS

Myth: We get 80 percent of our lifetime UV dose by the time we are eighteen years old.

Fact: This myth began in 1986 with publication of the theory that skin-cancer risk could be reduced later in life if sunscreen was applied during childhood. Even though the conclusion was theoretical and not based on scientific investigation, the so-called 80 percent rule is perpetuated time and again in medical and Internet settings. In 2003, an international team, including researchers from the U.S. Food and Drug Administration, finally evaluated actual lifetime exposure to UV radiation for a more accurate estimate. It turns out that less than 25 percent of our lifetime UV exposure is obtained by age eighteen. Writing in the Journal *Photochemistry and Photobiology* (2003), the researchers stated that UV exposure is fairly consistent over the course of a lifetime. This obviously means that protection against UV radiation should be a lifetime consideration.

Myth: Low SPF (sun protection factor) afforded by dietary interventions and in the 3 to 4 range is of little consequence to skin cancer and the prevention of skin aging.

Fact: Sadly, even some dermatologists scoff at low levels of SPF gained via dietary antioxidants. The dismissal of lifelong, low-level SPF protection as inconsequential reflects a lack of understanding of how SPF numbers are connected to skin-cancer risk. Even an SPF of 2 from fish oil or an SPF of 3 from dietary antioxidants (to say nothing of the synergy in a combination) would be associated with a major decrease in the risk of non-melanoma skin cancers. The reason is because of diminishing returns with each numerical SPF increase. An SPF of 2 blocks 50 percent of UVB radiation, while an SPF of 4 blocks 75 percent of radiation, and an SPF of 5 blocks 80 percent of the UV radiation. An SPF of 13 provides

only 13 percent more protection against UVB. Based on calcula-
tion, a dietary SPF of 4 would reduce the risk of non-melanoma
skin cancers by half or better over a lifetime. Clearly, that is
not inconsequential.

Finally, researchers from the Berlin Charité Hospital, led by skin-aging
expert and dermatology professor Juergen Lademann, reported that those
with higher dietary antioxidant intake via fruits and vegetables are much
less likely to present the visible signs of aging. The reports, in the German
trade journal *The Dermatologist* (2006), stated that the dietary habits of
those with a diet rich in colorful fruit and vegetables had the highest skin
levels of antioxidants, and this, in turn, translates into a more youthful
perceived age.

The researchers reported that vegetarians have higher levels of
antioxidants. In fact, studies show that vegetarians have significantly
higher levels of wrinkle-fighting carotenoids. These are an antioxidant
family found in high amounts in tomatoes, carrots, and peppers; one
particular carotenoid, lycopene, is a major defender against skin aging. In
fact, Lademann's group has recently shown that those with the highest skin
levels of lycopene have the lowest visible signs of aging.

YOUR SKIN, YOUNGER—WRINKLE PROTECTORS, WRINKLE PROMOTERS

The Monash University Study

After careful examination of the diets of 453 older adults from
Australia, Sweden, and Greece, researchers concluded that, in
addition to the usual suspects—sun and smoking—foods were
strongly linked to visible signs of aging. Some protectors and some
promoters emerged, as shown in this bulleted list.

Foods and Beverages Identified as Wrinkle Protectors

- Fatty fish rich in omega-3 fatty acids, such as sardines and anchovies
- Vegetables—in particular, dark green vegetables
- Whole-grain cereals
- Eggs
- Olive oil and monounsaturated fat
- Nuts and legumes
- Low-fat dairy, such as yogurt
- Tea and water
- Dark-colored fruits, such as cherries, prunes, apples
- Intake of zinc, a nutrient found in fish and seafood

Foods and Beverages Identified as Wrinkle Promoters

- Meats, in particular, processed meats
- High-fat dairy, such as ice cream
- White potatoes
- Butter and overall saturated fat
- Margarine
- Baked goods, such as cakes, pastries, and sugar-rich desserts
- Soft drinks

Emotional Connection and Stress Resiliency

Helle Rexbye, PhD, and colleagues from the University of Southern Denmark recently investigated additional lifestyle factors that may affect facial aging. The study, published in the journal *Age and Ageing* (2006), used data from almost two thousand older adult twins and determined once again the obvious connections to skin aging—sun and smoking. However, the researchers found other interesting and significant factors associated with facial wrinkling and looking older. Higher levels of day-to-day depressive symptoms, based on evaluations of factors such as well-being, energy levels, and mental focus, were associated with a more visually aged face. In fact, a woman with more depressive symptoms was perceived to be older by nearly half a decade.

Further evidence that stress contributes to looking old for one's age comes from a recent study in the journal *Plastic and Reconstructive Surgery* (2009). Here, researchers from Case Western Reserve University looked at almost two hundred pairs of identical twins. Once again, the results contradicted the notion that genetics explain our ability to defy aging skin. The usual suspects—smoking and sun—were both found to be age promoters in the twins who indulged the most. The unexpected finding was a stress connection. The twin who had a history of divorce was much more likely to be perceived as older. Furthermore, a history of using antidepressant drugs and greater alcohol use also resulted in a significantly older appearance.

> A healthy outlook can mean healthier skin.

In the Danish twin study by Rexbye, those with lower socioeconomic status (SES) were also more likely to experience wrinkles. While money can't buy happiness per se, it does provide security and, let's face it, those in the upper SES are unlikely to be holding down two minimum-wage jobs to make ends meet. Those residing in the higher SES are much more likely to engage in healthy lifestyle practices and have the means to afford quality health care, as well as preventive and healing interventions.

Those with higher SES are ultimately less likely to experience ill health through the aging process. Rates of depression, anxiety, reported chronic stress, and physical workload are higher in those with lower SES. Research shows that even though those with high SES might report high job strain, the folks with low SES and high job strain are much more likely to see consequential ill-health such as hypertension. The dietary choices of those with low SES deviate quite a bit from the wealthy, with much greater reliance on calorie-dense, nutrient-poor foods.

In sum, the research shows that chronic stress, depression, low mood states, and the associated health-compromising behaviors will influence the biological age of your face. Let's be honest: when you're under stress, how often do you reach for broccoli and Brussels sprouts? All of these factors are intertwined with the major physiological culprits in skin aging—inflammation and oxidative stress.

Stress promotes oxidative stress and inflammation, and poor dietary choices limit our ability to fight the inflammation and oxidative stress that promote skin aging. Indeed, poor dietary choices might limit our resiliency against stress, while additional environmental assaults dial up our requirement for more nutrients in skin-defense. The visible signs of aging then diminish well-being, self-esteem, and mental outlook, leading to more stress. The lack of control, the feeling that we can do nothing, will further compromise health-oriented behaviors. And so it goes—a never-ending downward cycle that will carry you face-first into skin aging. We will help you to stop this most vicious cycle at a number of different stages.

Modern Malnutrition

Let's discuss some harsh nutritional realities. Taking stock of our current nutritional intakes, the excesses and deficiencies, will help us understand where the voids are and how we can make changes for our skin. Currently, the North American diet is in a sorry state of affairs. Despite the abundance of calories, we are in many ways malnourished. The skin-aging process takes place in this dietary context.

WHOLE GRAINS

People may be trying to eat healthy. They may look for products with "whole grains" on the label, because fiber-rich whole grains are associated with sugar and insulin balance and greater satiety, as well as lower inflammatory chemicals in the body. Whole grains also contain antioxidant components within the fiber. Alas, the notion that the phrase "made with whole grains" on a box translates into a fiber-rich, low-sugar grain product isn't always true. You can find "made with whole grains" stamped on high-sugar cereals, for example. The molecular levels of whole grains used in these candy-like cereals may qualify for the self-designed corporate "made with whole grain" logo, yet it translates into a bowl full of 15 grams of sugar and only a single gram of fiber.

There is also a big difference between "100 percent whole grain," what the U.S. Food and Drug Administration (FDA) considers "whole grain," and what "made with whole grains" all mean in real terms. Of course 100 percent whole grain is, well, 100 percent whole grain. However, the FDA allows a product to be called whole grain if it is 51 percent whole grain by weight.

As for those clever "made with whole grains" marketing labels that are slapped on cereal-based products and baked goods, they're not worth the cardboard box they're written on. When you inventory the foods at your local convenience store, shopping centers, vending machines, schools, and on and on, you will find foods made with processed flour—with nutrients and fiber stripped away.

> The elimination of fiber from grain products is a big deal when it comes to preventing the skin's aging process, particularly because fiber-free carbohydrates cause elevations in blood sugar and insulin release.

SUGAR

Our overall intake of insulin-spiking, refined sugars has increased by eightfold over the past two hundred years. A massive increase in sugar intake has come from our fondness for high-fructose corn syrup (HFCS), as found in soft drinks. We increased our annual refined-sugar consumption from half of a pound per person, on average, in 1970 to more than 60 pounds per person by the late 1990s. Sugar encourages the production of skin-damaging molecules called Advanced Glycation End-products, aptly abbreviated as AGEs.

> The high sugars we consume, as well as the quantity of preformed AGEs in the foods we eat (because food preparation can make a huge difference in the direct AGE content of foods), are the nutritional equivalent of putting your face in front of a sunlamp.

FRUITS AND VEGGIES

Supported by volumes of research, government and private nutrition education groups encourage us to increase our intake of fruits and vegetables to ward off serious conditions like heart disease and cancer. Problem is, we aren't listening. We continue to shun fruits and vegetables.

More than 60 percent of Americans consume fast food on a regular basis, which translates into fewer colorful fruit-and-vegetable servings for adults and children alike.

The largest study to date, published in the *Journal of the American Dietetic Association* (2006), showed that, on average, we only consume a meager 1.5 servings daily of dark green and deeply colored orange or yellow vegetables. Take away potatoes, and only 29 percent of adults and 13 percent of children consume even the minimum recommended five servings of fruits and vegetables per day. Four foods account for half of total vegetable intake in U.S. adults—potatoes (mostly frozen and fried), iceberg lettuce, onions, and tomato. Let's state the obvious: this constitutes the trimmings on a burger and a side of fries!

If you need more evidence of our colorless, bland diets, consider a recent study in the *Journal of Cancer Education* (2007). Among more than 1,600 parents surveyed, not a single one consumed the five major dietary plant-color groups (reds, greens, orange-yellows, purple-blues, non-potato whites) on more than 3.5 days per week. Only 40 percent of parents and 26 percent of children ate from the five major color groups over the course of an entire week!

> A diet consistently rich in deeply colored plant foods provides a nutritional defense system for the skin. A steady diet devoid of colors opens up and exposes collagen and other skin structures to the ravages of aging.

WHAT MALNUTRITION MEANS FOR YOUR SKIN

Our paltry intake of fruits and vegetables and whole grains, and our complete lack of variety, ultimately translates into less skin protection. Currently at least half of the U.S. population does not meet the absolute minimum recommended dietary allowance (RDA) for skin-protective vitamins and minerals, including calcium, magnesium, zinc, and vitamin A and B family vitamins. In addition to the vitamins and minerals within unprocessed plant foods, these foods also contain more than twenty-five thousand micro-chemicals that give plants their color, taste, and texture.

These naturally occurring chemicals are called phytochemicals, and they include a mosaic of deeply colored plant pigments.

The colorful plant chemicals have, in turn, potent antioxidant activities. When you see the deep reds and purple colors of fresh blueberries, cherries, and beets; the deep greens in spinach and kale; and the oranges in carrots, you are staring phytochemicals in the face. Since there are so many different antioxidants and they work in synergy, much like an orchestra, it is important to obtain different dietary colors on a regular basis for full-spectrum protection.

Interestingly, plants produce phytochemicals as a defense mechanism for their own survival and health. This is precisely what consumption does for us as well: it supports our own defense mechanisms. While the bulk of scientific research on the *dietary* phytochemicals shows them to be protective against killers such as cardiovascular disease and various cancers, research also suggests their great potential in anti-aging. Note that we said dietary antioxidants; as we will discuss in chapter 2, the research supporting isolated antioxidants in pure chemical form has been falling flat on its face.

Essential Fats

Certain types of fats are essential to human life. "Essential" means we cannot make these special fats on our own, and in their absence, disease and ultimately death will follow. One of the first telltale signs of the lack of essential fatty acids (EFAs) is right on the skin. Lack of EFAs will manifest with dry, rough, and scaly skin.

THE FIRST ESSENTIAL FAT AND SKIN DISCOVERY

One might argue that St. Hilarion actually discovered the "essentiality" of dietary oil around 300 AD. He reportedly spent years in isolation, leading a voluntary monastic life sustained by a fat-free diet. His skin became dry, rough, and covered with scaly lesions—all of which were ameliorated when he incorporated oil into his diet.

Unsaturated fats were originally referred to as vitamin F to signify fat. In 1936, researchers showed that topical application of these EFAs could ameliorate the skin manifestations of dietary EFA deficiency. Following this, the U.S. Patent Office was filled with applications for a host of vitamin F–based skin creams, soaps, and other products.

Others, including Hugh Sinclair, MD, and colleagues at the University of Oxford, were showing that oral supplementation with EFAs could quickly reverse a deficiency and clear up skin problems. One particular area of interest was the EFA anti-aging potential in human skin. Sinclair reported in 1957 that an EFA deficiency worsened the skin-damaging influence of UV radiation and caused fragmentation of collagen, loss of dermal tissue, and reduced blood flow to the skin. In his landmark skin-nutrition review, published in the *Annales de la nutrition et de l'alimentation* (1957), this Oxford vice president lambasted the profession of dermatology for turning its back on the nutrition potential, referring to dermatology as a "backward branch of medicine." While other medical disciplines were starting to get into the trenches to truly investigate the relationship between diet and chronic diseases, dermatology was quickly tossing out all references to the lowly diet factor. But now dermatology is once again looking into the connection between nutrition and glowing skin.

OMEGA-3 ESSENTIAL FATTY ACIDS

Today North Americans' intake of omega-6 outnumbers omega-3 intake by a ratio as high as 20 to 1. This is an unacceptable ratio, one far removed from the ideal ratio of 2 to 1 (omega-6 to omega-3). There has been a massive decrease in the intake of omega-3 essential fatty acids over the past hundred years and a coincidental increase in the consumption of omega-6-rich vegetable oils (soybean, safflower, sunflower, and corn). Therefore, today we are faced not so much with an EFA deficiency, but rather with a specific omega-3 EFA deficiency.

While most of the foods we eat have omega-6 fatty acids, we need omega-3s for our skin because they provide insulation against UV damage and collagen destruction. Animals that are allowed to graze, to hunt and peck, or to forage have access to the naturally occurring omega-3 fatty acids in grasses, insects, and other natural sources. Try replacing some of your meats and eggs with free-range meats and omega-3 enriched eggs. You can also get your omega-3 supply from fish, seafood, nuts (especially walnuts), canola oil, flaxseeds, hemp, dark-green leafy vegetables, and even blueberries.

Dietary Fiber

In addition to the nutritional voids of vitamins and minerals, omega-3 fatty acids, and phytochemicals, the fourth pillar of inadequacy is that of dietary fiber. Since dietary fiber is found in unprocessed grains and whole fruits and vegetables, our fiber intake could be expected to be sub-par. North Americans typically consume only 13 grams of fiber per day—at least 33 percent less than was consumed with traditional diets a century ago. We should be consuming anywhere from 7 to 25 grams more, depending on our age and gender. Lack of dietary fiber speeds the release of sugar and insulin into the bloodstream. Over time, this may have serious collagen-damaging and inflammation-promoting implications in the dermis.

POST'S SKIN-FRIENDLY CEREALS

Sometimes finding a high-fiber, low-sugar cereal in the mass market can seem like a challenge. Here are our top four picks manufactured by Post, where "whole grain" on the label actually means whole grain in the box.

- Post Shredded Wheat 'n Bran: 57 grams of whole grain per serving.
- Post Shredded Wheat Original: 49 grams of whole grain per serving.
- Post Grape-Nuts Flakes: 23 grams of whole grain per serving.
- Post Bran Flakes: 16 grams of whole grain per serving.

Wisdom of the Dermatology Elders

Older dermatology textbooks, including the *Fundamentals of Medical Dermatology* (University of Pennsylvania, Department of Dermatology

Book Fund, 1942), recommended that patients with skin conditions substitute "whole wheat or graham bread or rolls for white flour products." The authors also advocated for "whole fruits" versus juices. Sixty-plus years before the U.S. government's 5-A-Day campaign for three servings of vegetables and two servings of fruits daily, dermatologists were advocating the consumption of "at least three vegetables and a salad a day" to promote healthy, youthful skin.

Old-school dermatology isn't a backward branch of medicine at all. Modern techniques to reduce the visible signs of aging—scalpel, botox, lasers, and other cutting-edge technologies—are not compatible with leprechaun-endorsed cereal and clown-endorsed fast food. It's time for us to return to our dermatological roots, time to delve deeper into the inside-out connection to skin health and its aging process. Our collagen, elastin, and stratum corneum cells are down on their knees begging for nutritional mercy.

2

Inflammation and Oxidative Stress: The Flames of Skin Aging

CHRONIC INFLAMMATION IS DRIVEN BY A number of factors, most notably a diet filled with the wrong types of fats and sugars—and its flip side, a diet devoid of healthy omega-3 fatty acids, dietary fiber, whole grains, and colorful fruits and vegetables. Throw in a chaser of psychological stress and physical exercise limited to changing the TV remote, and presto, you have an inflammatory assault on your skin.

Time magazine sometimes places a villain on its cover, and on February 23, 2004, that dishonor fell to chronic inflammation. Indeed, chronic inflammation earned its place in infamy because of its undeniable link to modern diseases such as heart disease, cancer, diabetes, and neurodegenerative diseases of the brain. Skin conditions are not immune to the ravages of inflammation. It is at the root of acne, psoriasis, and virtually all skin conditions in between. Inflammation also is at the root of skin aging, an inflammatory process that can be set in motion by both consistently poor dietary choices and chronic psychological stress. This is not the overt inflammation that plagues "-itis" conditions such as rheumatoid arthritis. Skin-aging inflammation is an insidious and subtle low-grade inflammation that damages skin in much the same way that waves erode a coastline. Once set in motion, inflammation in the skin will further promote oxidative stress.

Oxidative stress is a term that gets thrown around a lot these days. Let's step back for a moment to get a handle on what oxidative stress is all about. Skin is our great defender, the unsung hero that protects us from all sorts of assaults. One of the most identifiable enemies to human skin is the free radical, an agent that, when kept unchecked, will produce oxidative stress.

Free radicals are biological kleptomaniacs, and no amount of psychotherapy is going to quell their desire to steal. In the case of skin aging, they are taking electrons. When free radicals steal electrons from other molecules, the result is damage to delicate skin components and further inflammation. Inflammation promotes oxidative stress, and oxidative stress promotes inflammation in an ongoing vicious cycle.

Oxidative Stress: When oxygen is used to produce energy in the human body, one of the byproducts is the creation of highly reactive molecules called free radicals. They are highly reactive because each of them is an unpaired molecule looking for a partner. They can interact with and damage structural fats, proteins, and even delicate genetic components in a process called oxidative stress.

The generation of free radicals is never going to stop. And approximately 3 percent of oxygen used in the metabolic processes of our cells is converted to free radicals. So why bother to worry about skin aging? If we can't stop free radical production, how can we slow down skin aging and inflammation? The good news is that human skin has a wonderfully organized Department of Defense. It is equipped with two major systems that are capable of providing top-notch protection against free-radical damage:

1. Catalase, superoxide dismutase, and glutathione peroxidase—enzymes that race to neutralize free radicals.
2. Non-enzymatic antioxidant defense which directly uses vitamins and other nutrients—items like vitamins C and E, zinc, glutathione, and the so-called phytochemicals from plant-based foods and herbs.

One major caveat is that this wonderful antioxidant defense system depends entirely upon diet. Dietary nutrients turn on the ignition and ultimately drive the antioxidant enzymes, and the second line of defense, the non-enzymatic antioxidant armour, is obviously obtained directly through our foods and beverages of choice. Inflammation also can be dialed up or turned down by what we eat and drink.

The other major caveat is that the antioxidant defense system loses its efficiency through the aging process, and there is also an increased propensity to produce inflammatory chemicals in the skin as we age. That doesn't mean that the young are immune; however, it does mean that inappropriate dietary choices made by older adults, those who pull up often to the drive-through window of major fast-food chains, will have massive skin-compromising consequences.

MELANOMA EPIDEMIC

Melanoma rates are increasing at an astonishing rate worldwide, with a 24 percent increase in Israel in 2006 alone. In Japan the rates have been steadily climbing since the 1990s. In the United Kingdom the rates have doubled in the last six years. Ireland has seen an 84 percent increase in malignant melanoma among males over the last decade. Even India, which has had relatively low levels of melanoma, is observing an increase. The United States has also had a marked increase over the last twenty years, particularly in the young.

As much as the media and some dermatologists like to point to tanning beds, it is a far stretch to place the sole blame on these machines. Research certainly indicates they can contribute to the skin aging process—decreasing skin firmness and elasticity. We strongly urge against the use of these machines. However, population studies and the largest review to date in the journal Photodermatology, Photoimmunology & Photomedicine (2007) have not made convincing associations between sun-bed use and melanoma risk. While these tanning beds may damage the skin and increase the risk of non-melanoma skin cancer among the small percentage of the population who use them regularly (less than 10 percent of adults), it appears there are other environmental factors at play with the sudden rise in melanoma. We cannot write off this epidemic to a thinned-out ozone layer exposing us to more UV radiation—the ozone layer has been improving for well over a decade now. Some researchers, including Dr. Orjan Hallberg of Sweden, have been postulating that exposure to electromagnetic frequencies (EMF) via wireless phones, computers, and the like could be helping to drive the higher melanoma rates. He made a strong argument in the European Journal of Cancer Prevention (2008), showing that it is the ability of EMF to compromise the immune-repair systems in the skin that can increase skin cancer risk. The studies on cellular phone EMF exposure to animals supports his theory, as does a specific increase in the rates of facial melanoma in young adults since 2000. A stunning new study in the Journal of Toxicology and Environmental Health (2009) shows that mobile phone radiation has a synergistic effect in cellular disturbances when combined with other EMF (see Is Your Cell Phone Wrinkling Your Skin? on page 113).

How Fat-Induced Inflammation Produces Wrinkles

By looking a little deeper at how inflammatory chemicals are actually produced in the skin, we can make it easier to see how simple dietary changes can make such a big difference. One major class of inflammatory chemicals produced in the skin, the very ones that cause damage to collagen, is called the prostaglandins. The chief offender among the prostaglandins is called PGE2. While other inflammatory chemicals exist, we will focus on PGE2 because it has been consistently linked to skin aging.

PGE2: An inflammatory chemical that is linked to aging and is turned on by UV rays and excess vegetable oils.

This nasty character turns on those matrix metalloproteinases (MMPs) we talked about—the enzymes that damage and fragment your collagen. PGE2 also inhibits the formation or production of new collagen by our fibroblasts. Clearly, PGE2 is a "worst-case scenario" chemical for aging skin. It breaks up and shatters our otherwise well-organized collagen while turning off the valve of the fibroblast pipeline so that no new collagen can be formed.

Ultraviolet rays have been shown to increase PGE2 production in the skin. In particular UVA (the aging one) is a major offender in turning up the inflammatory PGE2 levels in the dermis.

However, UV rays are not the whole story. PGE2 levels can be introduced into the skin in other ways, not the least of which is through our dietary fats. An excess of linoleic-acid-rich vegetable oils—most notably corn, soybean, sunflower, and safflower oil—can elevate the production of PGE2, which is a major driving force in inflammation. The reason is because the linoleic acid found in the aforementioned oils provides the raw material for the manufacture of PGE2. Don't think for a moment that dietary fats, when orally consumed, have no influence on the far reaches of the skin and its inflammatory chemicals. They can—and they do.

THE SKIN NEEDS AN OIL CHANGE

Edward Pinckney, MD, reported in 1973 that among more than one thousand patients evaluated at a plastic surgeon's office over two years, those with the greatest consumption of polyunsaturated oils had the most visible signs of premature aging. The evaluation assessed skin elasticity, wrinkles, skin tone, and other visible signs of aging. The results were then matched with estimates of polyunsaturated oil intake.

In the 1980s, researchers from Baylor College of Medicine discovered a two-and-a-half-fold difference in the dermal levels of PGE2 in animals fed chow where the fat source was a linoleic-acid-rich corn oil diet versus those with fish oil as a fat source.

North Americans today have a massive annual intake of vegetable oils, three times more per person than in 1960. If the production of PGE2 within the skin remains consistently elevated, it will take its toll on collagen.

Using Fats to Fight Inflammation

Going back to the 1930s, some medical doctors who lived with the Canadian Inuits observed that the Inuits' skin was unblemished and youthful. The first report was by Israel Rabinowitch, MD, DSc, of McGill University who spent months with the Inuit of Hudson Bay in 1935. Others, including Otto Schaefer, MD, who spent three decades treating the Inuit in Northwestern Canada, noted higher rates of acne and an assault to healthy skin as Western dietary influences encroached. Those dietary influences were the mountains of sugar, processed carbohydrates, and unhealthy fats we hauled into the Inuit pantries.

What Westerners removed from the Inuits was a traditional diet high in anti-inflammatory omega-3 fatty acids, as well as fiber and antioxidants. One skin-protecting component was far and away higher in the traditional diets of isolated communities—omega-3 fatty acids. As the research would later show, the anti-inflammatory properties of omega-3 fatty acids were the cornerstone of the skin-healthy, traditional Inuit diet. The story of cod-liver oil provides the link between the traditional Inuit diet and our modern-day knowledge of omega-3.

Cod-liver oil was introduced to the masses during the 1930s, when the scientific interest and commercial marketing surrounding the oil was based solely on its vitamin A and D content. The fact that cod-liver oil contained important omega-3 fatty acids was a non-issue for decades. In the late 1950s, researchers began reporting that oral cod-liver oil was working wonders for arthritis. Some European rheumatologists even reported anti-inflammatory benefit when they injected cod-liver oil into the joints.

Around the same time, a small group of dermatologists were writing up cases of marked improvement in inflammatory skin conditions when specially prepared cod-liver oil ointments and lotions were applied to the skin. Despite the reported value, these lotions never really took off in the marketplace, likely because cod-liver oil has a distinct fishy smell (a delicate way of saying the liver oil reeks to the high heavens).

Still, these publications finally fueled researchers to think beyond vitamins A and D. As good as these vitamins are for skin, there had to be more to cod-liver oil's benefits. As scientists began to learn more about omega-3 fatty acids in the 1970s, researchers from the department of dermatology at Copenhagen's famed Finsen Institute made an important observation. Niels Kromann, MD, and colleagues reported that the Greenland Inuit had very low rates of psoriasis and other skin diseases. The Danish researchers also reported one major new finding: despite the same magnitude of UV exposure, the Greenland Inuit had rates of skin cancer that were far lower than would be expected for others in Northwest Europe. Could the omega-3 fatty acids be the UV-protecting factor? Investigations into the skin-specific anti-inflammatory and UV-protecting properties of omega-3 fatty acids would follow shortly thereafter.

The experimental and population studies started to show a clear pattern—all polyunsaturated fatty acids could not be painted with the same brush. Fish oil, rich in eicosapentaenoic acid (EPA), an omega-3 fatty acid, was proving to be protective against UV-induced skin cancer. Chemical markers in the skin that are known to be associated with high skin-cancer risk were ten times lower in animals fed fish oil versus those fed omega-6 corn oil. Supplementation with fish oil also proved to lower that age-inducing chemical feared by any living strand of collagen—yes, PGE2.

Even when animals were provided with just enough omega-6 linoleic acid to meet essential-fatty-acid requirements, researchers observed a threefold reduction in PGE2 levels when fish oil was added to the mix. Remember, the greater the omega-6 vegetable oil intake, the higher the PGE2 levels, unless they are held in check by fish oil. The epidemiological, or population studies, supported the initial observation of the Inuit—higher omega-3 intake and more fish and seafood in the diet go hand in hand with a significantly reduced risk of various skin cancers.

These experimental and population studies were interesting, yet we needed more. As the saying in science goes, correlation does not equal causation. In other words, associations are just that, associations. Until someone actually used fish oil in humans, the connection would remain speculative.

The folks from Baylor College of Medicine changed that with a publication in the *Archives of Dermatological Research* (1992). They reported that the oral administration of fish oil (2.8 grams of EPA daily) limited the influence of UV radiation in adults. The fish oil was estimated to provide an SPF of 1.15. While that might sound like a joke, an incredibly small number compared to that listed on your Coppertone bottle, a consistent daily SPF of 1.15 actually translates to a 30 percent reduction in the lifetime risk of skin cancer. For our purposes, since agents that reduce skin cancer are typically anti-aging for the skin, the finding showed the potential of fish oil for the maintenance of youthful skin.

Follow-up studies by other groups have also found that omega-3 fish-oil supplementation protects against UV-induced skin damage and keeps PGE2 in check. In addition, the more recent studies have answered a lingering question: do omega-3 fatty acids like EPA actually increase in skin tissue when orally supplemented? The answer is a clear yes; in fact, 4 grams of EPA taken orally for twelve weeks resulted in eightfold higher levels of EPA when human skin was subjected to biopsy.

New studies from the United Kingdom have shown that orally consumed fish oil may not only reduce the redness and skin cell damage that occurs with UV exposure, but also work to protect the delicate DNA within skin cells. There have been other equally exciting developments related to topically applied EPA in sun protection and collagen support; thankfully, new deodorization technology has succeeded in removing the fishy smell to allow for commercial use of topical EPA. We will talk more about that in chapter 7.

Omega-3 and Elasticity

The benefits of omega-3 fatty acids in human skin don't end with collagen protection and limitation of UV damage. Since EPA has been proven to build up in human skin tissue, there are additional structural benefits. For example, fish oil can improve the elasticity of blood vessels. In the absence of omega-3 fatty acids, our blood vessel walls become stiff and blood flow is compromised. It may be a similar situation in our skin. While we still don't know for sure, the incorporation of omega-3 fatty acids into the skin area over time likely makes skin cells themselves more flexible. A study in the *Journal of Dermatological Research* (2008) did show an improvement in skin elasticity among women taking just over 1 gram of EPA-rich fish oil for three months.

FISHY MYTHS AND MISCONCEPTIONS

Research has supported the original advice of cosmetic dermatologist Irwin Lubowe, MD, who recommended fish and seafood for their skin anti-aging properties in the 1970s. Since we also advocate for fish consumption, we think it is important to clear up the controversy and widespread misinformation that exists in books and Internet sources.

1. **What are the best sources of omega-3 fatty acids?** Oily fish including salmon, sardines, anchovies, and mackerel are very high in the dermal-protecting, anti-inflammatory omega-3 fats called eicosapentaenoic acid (EPA) and docosahexaenoic acid (DHA).

2. **Are these fish safe? Aren't they high in mercury?** None of the fish listed above are high in mercury. Contrary to popular opinion, the mercury in both farmed and wild salmon is negligible. Farmed salmon is, however, high in toxic environmental chemicals called polychlorinated biphenyl compounds (PCBs) that have been linked to cancer and cognitive dysfunction. You don't need to shop at high-end gourmet shops to buy wild salmon. Most canned salmon is, in fact, wild Canadian and Alaskan salmon. Check the label for the wild-source logo.

3. **So what fish are high in mercury?** Fresh tuna sushi or sashimi, tuna steaks, swordfish, shark, and tilefish are at the top of the list. However, new data from the U.S. Food and Drug Administration suggest that grouper, sea trout, orange roughy, and bluefish are all fish of concern. When it comes to canned tuna, the more expensive version, white albacore, has higher levels of mercury than previously thought. The chunk light is low in mercury and more acceptable for regular consumption. For more details and a tuna calculator based on weight and gender, go to the Environmental Working Group's website at http://www.ewg.org.

4. **Is farmed fish a source of the linoleic acid we are over-consuming?** Yes! Farmed salmon, tilapia, and catfish contain significant amounts of the linoleic acid that can drive inflammation. Linoleic acid is virtually absent from wild sources.

5. **Is it possible to reduce environmental toxins through cooking?** Research has shown that up to 50 percent of PCBs can be reduced through various cooking methods and with removal of the skin from fish. Unfortunately, the opposite is true of mercury. With cooking, the mercury remains behind, leading to concentrations per weight that are 45 percent higher than in raw fish. The result is even worse when fish are breaded in oil, which can lead to mercury levels more than 70 percent higher than in raw fish.

6. **What about fish-oil supplements and contaminants?** Published research from Harvard Medical School and independent testing by Consumer Reports and ConsumerLab.com have all concluded that commercially available fish-oil supplements are generally free of environmental contaminants such as mercury and PCBs. You may also want to check out the Canadian International Fish Oil Standards program (http://www.ifosprogram.com), which independently tests fish-oil supplements for quality and names brands on its website.

7. **In the final analysis, do the benefits of fish intake outweigh risks?** Yes! After extensive review, researchers from Harvard's School of Public Health reported in the *Journal of the American Medical Association* (2006) that the benefits of fish intake do exceed the potential risks. The researchers advised sidestepping high-mercury fish and consuming a wide variety of fish and seafood to minimize risk.

SOURCES OF EPA AND DHA

Fish/Seafood	Total EPA/DHA (mg/100g)
Mackerel	2300
Chinook salmon	1900
Herring	1700
Anchovy	1400
Sardine	1400
Coho Salmon	1200
Trout	600
Spiny lobster	500
Halibut	400
Shrimp	300
Catfish	300
Sole	200
Cod	200

OMEGA-6 AND OMEGA-3
CONTENT (%) OF DIETARY OILS

Oil	Omega-6	Omega-3
Safflower	75	0
Sunflower	65	0
Corn	54	0
Cottonseed	50	0
Sesame	42	0
Peanut	32	0
Soybean	51	7
Canola	20	9
Walnut	52	10
Flax	14	57

The "Good" Omega-6

If you have strolled through the supplement aisle of your local pharmacy or health-food store, you may have noticed lots of essential-fatty-acid supplements that list omega-6 in the ingredients—products with omega-3-6-9, or even omega-3-6-7-9. Because your authors have just warned of the numerous health consequences of taking too much omega-6, why on earth would products with omega-6 be sold in plain view? The answer is simple: the omega-6 in such products is the "good" omega-6, or more specifically, gamma-linolenic acid (GLA). GLA is typically derived from borage, evening primrose, or black-currant seed oils. Since borage contains the highest amount of GLA per gram (about 20 percent), it is often the oil of choice.

GLA slows down the manufacture of collagen-busting, skin-inflaming PGE2. It's a similar story to that of EPA from fish oil. Since GLA and fish oil use different mechanisms to limit PGE2 production, it makes perfect sense that research shows these oils to have synergistic properties.

Studies show what you can do with GLAs:

- Try supplementing with evening primrose oil (containing approximately 400 milligrams of GLA) for three months or longer. Evening primrose has been shown to improve skin smoothness significantly. Major improvements in the condition of the skin were noted after just one month!
- Consume approximately 500 milligrams of GLA from borage oil. This helps with hydration: it's been found to reduce water loss through the epidermis significantly after two months of use. It's also been found to alleviate dry skin and itchy skin, which makes sense if the skin becomes more hydrated.
- Keep taking that GLA! Not only does oral GLA decrease water loss from the skin and improve overall hydration, but it also significantly improves firmness, roughness, elasticity, and resistance to fatigue.
- Try combining fish oil and GLA from borage. This will significantly improve skin hydration, and you'll reduce the amount of water lost through the epidermis. You might also find that roughness and scaling of the skin are reduced.

- Try a yogurt drink or probiotic with borage oil. In addition to improving the stratum corneum barrier, absorption of GLA is almost doubled when taken with yogurt!

While you may be pleasantly surprised by short-term omega-3 and GLA supplementation, don't expect results until after a few weeks. The epidermis needs at least a month or more to turn itself over, and since oral EFA supplements can take twenty-one days or so before any significant elevations are noted, results can sometimes take months. Most often, the results are well worth the wait. Let's sum up by stating clearly that consuming essential fatty acids, EPA and GLA in particular, is a major step to maintaining youthful, smooth, and well-hydrated skin. EPA and GLA are cornerstones in the new inside-out science of nutritional dermatology.

IRWIN I. LUBOWE, MD: GIVING A PIONEER CREDIT WHEN CREDIT IS DUE

The first dermatologist to recommend a diet heavy in oily fish and seafood, as well as oral antioxidant supplements, was Irwin Lubowe, MD. He was a clinical professor of dermatology at New York Medical College and author of several books including *New Hope for Your Skin.* In the late 1970s, he was at the cutting edge of nutritional dermatology, advocating for B vitamins, calcium, magnesium, zinc, and vitamin D for the prevention of aging skin. He also recommended oral intake of superoxide dismutase (SOD), an enzyme preparation the Japanese had been using as an internal antioxidant.

Writing in the *Journal of Applied Nutrition* (1979), he recommended sardines, shellfish, salmon, tuna, trout, flounder, scrod, bass, and halibut for the prevention of skin aging. Before fish oil was in vogue, he intended to provide structural building blocks for skin. He also developed a cream to help with skin firming. He reported that his patients not only witnessed an improvement in the visible signs of aging after eight weeks on this regimen but also reported an improved mental outlook.

At the time, this type of intervention was novel, and critics were many, with one dermatologist stating in 1985, "A New York dermatologist, Dr. Lubowe, is equally outlandish in holding out hope for reversing the ravages of age by modern scientific discoveries." The critic then went on to dismiss the benefits of SOD. Yet, over the years, oral and topical SOD has been shown to decrease inflammation and improve skin appearance. Unfortunately, Lubowe died in 1989, more than a decade before dermatologists once again began advocating a high fish and antioxidant-supplemented diet for the prevention of aging skin.

Antioxidants to the Rescue

At the beginning of this chapter, we discussed oxidative stress and how free-radical generation, if left unchallenged, can be a massive contributor to the skin-aging process. Since the antioxidant defense systems in the skin depend entirely on nutrition for their operations, it's important to pay attention to your diet and take oral supplemental antioxidants for UV protection and anti-aging. But research behind isolated antioxidants such as vitamin E or vitamin C alone has largely been disappointing. As our knowledge of antioxidants expands, we have become aware that certain antioxidants offer exceptional skin-protecting properties when allowed to work with other antioxidants.

The ACE Card—Three Key Vitamins

Vitamin A has been considered a great friend to healthy skin for many decades. In the 1930s, researchers first reported that vitamin A supplementation could prevent dry, flaky, and scaly skin. In 1942, the first reports showing anti-acne properties of vitamin A were published.

MORE INSPIRATION FROM THE INUIT

The backdrop to the investigations of vitamin A for skin was, once again, the Inuit diet. Jon Straumfjord, MD, was the first researcher to show that acne can be significantly improved with vitamin A supplements. He wrote in the journal *Northwest Medicine* (1943) that "the acne-free Inuit who lives after the manner of his father not only ingests much fat but also consumes 50,000 international units (IUs) of vitamin A daily." Straumfjord began using halibut-liver oil, a supplement high in both vitamin A and—although he didn't know it at the time—omega-3 fatty acids for acne patients. His results showed marked improvement in the course of patients' acne when it was treated with the oil.

Not only will vitamin A help with acne and getting rid of dry, scaly skin, but it also fights free radicals and protects against the classic redness of sunburn. You can take vitamin A as an oral supplement, topically, or through diet by making sure you have foods rich in vitamin A in your everyday diet. Retinol has emerged as a topical vitamin A skin-care star.

Vitamin C has specific skin-structure importance, but its levels decline through the aging process. In 1949, vitamin C was shown to be essential for the manufacture and maintenance of collagen. Vitamin C protects collagen and maintains its structure via the vitamin's strong antioxidant activities in the skin. In the process of defending us against UV and other environmental assaults, vitamin C is depleted from our skin, which is why levels decrease as we age. Like vitamin A, vitamin C reduces sunburn and potential sun-induced skin damage, and it has been shown to protect against UV-induced skin cancer in animals.

Our stratum corneum is particularly rich in the third member of the ACE antioxidant vitamins—fat-soluble vitamin E. Vitamin E helps various inflammatory dermatological skin conditions and is critical in the development of normal, well-functioning collagen, which explains its wound-healing properties. Furthermore, dietary vitamin E protects lipid, or fat, components of the skin when subjected to UV radiation.

We know each dietary ACE vitamin has UV-protecting properties and may even reduce the risk of skin cancers. So what happens when we orally consume ACE vitamins? Unfortunately, research has shown that taking these antioxidants separately will have no positive influence on your skin. The key is synergy. Combined vitamins C, E, and beta-carotene (vitamin A) offer UV protection. Specifically, studies show that taking oral vitamin C (about 2 grams), vitamin E (between 500 and 1000 IUs), and vitamin A family carotenoids (25 milligrams) for several weeks will significantly lower sunburn response to UV radiation in humans. Remember: what you eat is important and directly affects your skin. Those studies indicate that synergy of dietary antioxidants is what gives colorful fruits and vegetables the edge.

> Take ACE vitamins together as oral supplements, or eat them together by consuming colorful fruits and vegetables.

In fact, taking individual antioxidants in supplement form can have a dark side. Taken alone at high levels, these vitamins may actually act as pro-oxidants—yes, the very opposite of antioxidant protection. The precise reason why isolated antioxidants turn rogue and become pro-oxidants remains unclear. There are lots of theories. However, the most common theories revolve around the fact that antioxidants work like an orchestra. When you start taking very high doses of vitamin C or E alone, you mess around with the sounds of the orchestra.

A number of studies have indicated that beta-carotene taken alone as a supplement may act as a pro-oxidant in a way that actually promotes cancer in smokers. Vitamin E taken alone has been associated with increased risk of dying an earlier death, and vitamin C supplements (not dietary vitamin C) taken alone increase the risk of cardiovascular disease in women with diabetes.

The good news is that taking antioxidants together can negate the potential pro-oxidant effects of individual antioxidants. When antioxidants are drawn from foods and taken in the diet, the full orchestra covers up the small pro-oxidant mistake of one member. When you take antioxidants together, your skin cells will be thrilled with the results.

FEED YOUR SKIN: HIGHEST ANTIOXIDANT-RICH FOODS

- Acai
- Alfalfa
- Apple vinegar
- Applesauce
- Artichoke
- Asparagus
- Avocado
- Basil
- Beans (red, pinto, black, navy)
- Beets
- Bell peppers
- Black pepper
- Blackberry
- Black-eyed peas
- Blueberry
- Broccoli
- Brussels sprouts
- Cherries
- Chili powder
- Cilantro
- Cinnamon
- Cloves
- Cocoa
- Cranberry
- Dates
- Eggplant
- Elderberry
- Figs
- Fuji Apples
- Ginger
- Green tea
- Kale
- Nuts (all are high, walnuts in particular)
- Oatmeal and whole-grain breakfast cereals
- Olive oil, high-quality
- Oranges
- Oregano
- Parsley
- Peaches
- Pears
- Plums
- Pomegranate
- Prunes
- Purple cauliflower
- Purple sweet potato

- Raspberry
- Red cabbage
- Red grapes
- Red-leaf lettuce
- Red potatoes
- Spinach
- Strawberry
- Tangerines
- Turmeric

Food-Based UV Protection for Your Skin

Once researchers started uncovering the synergy of food-based antioxidants for skin health, the focus turned to other nonvitamin antioxidants that could serve as UV protectors. Those amazing phytochemicals we consume in healthy foods and beverages have skin-protecting and age-proofing nutrients. A diet rich in a variety of colorful fruits and vegetables can put the brakes on the skin-aging process. Here's what you should eat:

FOODS WITH LYCOPENE

A member of the vitamin A family of antioxidants called carotenoids, lycopene is one antioxidant that has UV-protecting properties. It has been shown to prevent UV-induced sunburn. Lycopene is abundant in tomato products and also found in apricot, pink grapefruit, guava, watermelon, and if you can find them, red carrots.

The most interesting study compared a lycopene juice, a tomato paste, a supplement tomato extract with lycopene, and a synthetic lycopene supplement. After twelve weeks of consumption, all groups except the synthetic lycopene consumers had significant reductions in sunburn after experimental UV exposure. The results showed that the adults consuming 5 to 10 milligrams of lycopene had an almost 50 percent decrease in the sunburn reaction.

This is yet another study underscoring the notion that whole foods or food-based supplements are much more likely to make a difference than synthetic supplements. When you decide to incorporate lycopene in your diet, consider tomatoes or a tomato-extract supplement and steer clear of synthetic lycopene. Topical lycopene, as we will discuss in chapter 7, can also provide skin support and UV protection.

COCOA

Generally speaking, dietary items that are heart-healthy are also skin-healthy. We have already seen this with omega-3 fatty acids, and the cocoa story provides another excellent example. Over the last decade, researchers have been looking into the heart-healthy properties of dark chocolate, or more specifically, its cocoa. Cocoa can improve blood flow in arteries and reduce blood pressure and cholesterol. Very importantly, cocoa has been shown to have strong anti-inflammatory and antioxidant properties.

Just like tomato-based products, cocoa helps protect against UV radiation. It also helps improve dry skin, skin thickness (remember that the dermis thins out through the aging process), and scaling. One important caveat, and it's a big one—a low dose of cocoa antioxidants, the level you might find in a milk chocolate bar, offers no UV protection, skin hydrating, or other objective benefits.

THE COCOA CONNECTION

The *Journal of Nutrition* (2006) published a study showing that consuming a drink that contained 329 milligrams of cocoa antioxidants (flavonols) reduced sunburn for otherwise healthy middle-aged women when they were exposed to UV radiation. In addition to the UV protective properties of cocoa, the researchers found that consuming the 329 milligrams of cocoa antioxidants daily for three months improved skin hydration and skin thickness, and decreased roughness and scaling of the skin.

The researchers followed up with a second study in the *European Journal of Nutrition* (2006) that looked for more immediate benefit to the skin when high-antioxidant cocoa is ingested. This time, they found that consuming 329 milligrams of cocoa flavonols significantly improved blood flow to the dermis. In fact, blood flow to the skin increased by almost twofold within two hours of the cocoa being ingested.

This was a golden discovery within nutritional dermatology, a ground-breaking piece of research when you consider that aging skin is crying out for a twofold increase in nutrient-dense blood to a dermis starved of nutrients and antioxidants. You can think of the cocoa as a direct supplier of its own antioxidants and as a carrier for all antioxidants delivered to the dermis because of the cocoa's ability to improve blood flow. Scientists have also reported that topical application of naturally occurring cocoa chemicals can improve aspects of skin aging.

GREEN TEA

This is yet another antioxidant-rich item for healthy, glowing skin that was inspired by cardiovascular research. Green tea contains important antioxidants and anti-inflammatory chemicals. More than two dozen studies have shown that green tea's antioxidants—and its component epigallocatechin-3-gallate (EGCG), in particular—can help prevent UV-induced skin cancer and DNA damage. While more human data is needed, the largest review to date, published in *Photodermatology, Photoimmunology & Photomedicine* (2007) concluded that "the available evidence indicates that green tea has many biological effects that ameliorate the damaging effects of both UVA and UVB radiation."

In addition to providing UV protection, a topical and oral green-tea supplement combination, administered for eight weeks, has been shown to improve the dermal elastic tissue in healthy women with moderately aged skin. Other teas from the same plant (*Camellia sinensis*), including white tea, oolong tea, and even black tea, are being investigated for protection against UV damage and overall promotion of healthy skin. In addition, South African rooibos tea has been in the spotlight recently for its ability to lower inflammation and protect against skin cancer.

GREEN TEA—PROS AND A CON

With their collagen-protecting properties, the antioxidants within green tea (particularly the natural EGCG chemical) may indeed be the skin's best friend. These days you don't have to hunt too far to find green tea products. However, not all green tea is alike, and when it comes to skin protection, many of these beverages are nutritional wolves in sheep clothing.

The highest grade of green tea is Japanese *matcha*—a fine powder of green tea leaves. Matcha green tea is grown under specific conditions, including avoidance of direct sunlight on the leaves. In 2003, researchers from the University of Colorado found that the concentration of EGCG available from drinking matcha is up to 137 times greater than the amount of EGCG available from other commercially available green teas. Packaged matcha and other high-grade green teas (loose and bagged) from Japan are available at http://www.kenkonutrition.com.

At the lowest end of the antioxidant scale, we have the convenience store fridge and vending machine bottled variety. Sadly, most of the high-sugar (some have as much as 42 grams of sugar!) or artificially sweetened drinks are nothing more than water with a few molecules of actual green tea. Despite the fancy antioxidant logos, the USDA assays found less than 4 milligrams of EGCG in bottled tea. Researchers from Oregon State University recently reported that freshly brewed green tea had up to 100 times more antioxidants than the mass-market bottles assayed.

In the interest of your collagen, keep moving past these bottles of sugar water disguised as green tea. Here's a tip: if you want the convenience and portability of a pre-made green tea, consider the Ito En brand. The Japanese company has introduced a number of unsweetened or very slightly sweetened green teas, including the *Sencha Shot* which delivers 152 milligrams of EGCG per small 6.4-ounce can and can be found at http://www.itoen.com.

COFFEE

For years coffee has had an unjustified reputation as a dietary villain. In truth, it is one of the most significant sources of dietary antioxidants in the North American diet, and a growing body of research is turning around the common notion that coffee is bad. Coffee drinking has been associated with a 30 percent decrease in the risk of diabetes, and lifetime consumption is associated with a decreased risk of cognitive decline later in life, as well as a decreased risk of liver disease, colon cancer, and gallstones. Some questions have been raised concerning osteoporosis; however, as long as a coffee drinker meets daily calcium requirements, the coffee appears to have no detrimental influence on his or her bone health. One caveat with coffee—don't make a habit of drinking it on an empty stomach. Despite the overall benefits and apparent protective properties in the prevention of diabetes, Canadian research indicates that caffeinated (versus decaf) coffee an hour before breakfast can increase blood sugar levels by 250 percent! Best to drink it with or following a meal.

With regard to the skin, a report in the *European Journal of Cancer Prevention* (2007) indicates that regular coffee consumption can reduce the risk of non-melanoma skin cancer by up to 36 percent. Components of raw coffee beans have been shown recently to double the production of the critically important dermal collagen, elastin, and GAGs. Look for extracts of raw coffee beans to become an exciting new ingredient in topical skin care.

GREEN VEGETABLES

While fresh iceberg lettuce may give sandwiches and salads a certain crunchy appeal, it is not a nutritional powerhouse. The giveaway is in its name "iceberg," implying water with a slight hint of green. Remove this "vegetable" from the stats, and North American green-vegetable consumption plummets to fractional amounts in the total diet. We seem to have an aversion to deeply colored green foods, which is a shame because they can be very beneficial for our skin.

Those deep-green leafy vegetables contain an important, skin-friendly antioxidant called lutein, which will help fight free radicals that damage your skin and give you UV protection. While the carotenoid antioxidant family is most often associated with red foods, it also shows up in deep green plants. There is an abundance of lutein in kale, broccoli, spinach, watercress, parsley, and basil. Zeaxanthin, another carotenoid antioxidant with skin-friendly properties, shows up in yellow-orange foods such as corn and orange peppers. Both lutein and zeaxanthin can be found in the yolk of free-range eggs as well.

In 2002, Italian researchers showed that 6 milligrams of lutein and 0.3 milligrams of zeaxanthin reduced UV damage in humans. In particular, the antioxidant combination protected the lipid components of skin from damage. More recently, the same Italian group reported on a three-month study using 10 milligrams of lutein and 0.6 milligrams of zeaxanthin. The results, published in the journal *Skin Pharmacology & Physiology* (2007), showed that, taken orally, the combination significantly improved skin elasticity.

Lutein and zeaxanthin together also improved the skin barrier and hydration, probably because they prevented damage to the lipids in the stratum corneum. All of these parameters were enhanced when the oral supplement was administered at the same time as a topical preparation containing lutein and zeaxanthin. This is the new direction in dermatology—inside-out and outside-in working together to improve the health and appearance of skin in the presence of environmental assaults.

There is one more important reason to consume liberal amounts of dark-green vegetables as part of your skin-healthy diet: they are alkaline, and the pH of your body is important in skin health as well. The connection between our current overconsumption of acidic foods and the promotion of visible signs of aging is fully discussed in chapter 7: Skin Food II, our dietary supplement chapter.

SOY FOODS

Part of the legume family, the soybean has been a staple in Asian cooking for five thousand years. The lowly legume is at the top of the list of foods that may have wrinkle-protecting properties. Soybeans are rather unique due to their high concentration of important phytochemicals, a family of antioxidants called flavonoids. After being ingested, soybean flavones are broken down by our gut bacteria to release active daidzein and genistein, chemicals with antioxidant and anti-inflammatory properties.

> Most of the research on soybeans for human health has focused on cardiovascular disease. Indeed, the soybean is one of the few foods for which the U.S. Food and Drug Administration has allowed a specific health claim, based on soy's heart-healthy properties.

The antioxidant and anti-inflammatory properties of daidzein and genistein offer significant protection to skin cells. Recently, research has shown that oral soybean-antioxidants reach the skin from the inside to improve skin elasticity. Topical, or external, administration of soy antioxidants can improve dermal structure, protect collagen, and increase production of the skin's scaffolding—the glycosaminoglycans (GAGs). Topical soybean-antioxidant extracts also may help prevent UV-induced damage and delay the aging process in the skin.

> A 2006 study showed that the average daily intake of soy antioxidants in Japan was 25 to 50 milligrams per day, largely from tofu, soy milk, natto, miso, tempeh, and soy sauce. North Americans consume less than 20 milligrams of these antioxidants over the course of a week.

Note that the fermented forms of soy—natto, miso, soy sauce—are the emerging stars of the soy family. Research shows that daidzein and genistein are absorbed more easily from fermented soy, and in head-to-head studies, fermented soy seemed to protect against cancer, rather than the unfermented soy found in soy ice cream, tofu, soy burgers, and soy shakes.

Dark Red-Purple Foods

More than a dozen years ago, Italian researchers first found that red (or blood) oranges might have sunburn-protecting properties in humans. Since then, a host of experimental studies have shown that the dark red and purple pigments in fruits and vegetables may offer significant protection to skin cells. These deeply colored pigments are called anthocyanins, and they are found in abundance in blueberries, blackberries, pomegranates, cherries, purple sweet potatoes, dark grapes, red cabbage, purple cauliflower, chokeberry, purple carrots, purple corn, and, of course, blood oranges.

Higher consumption of dietary anthocyanins is associated with lower risk of cardiovascular disease, diabetes, arthritis, and various cancers. The reason, once again, is almost certainly due to the strong antioxidant and anti-inflammatory activities of these colorful chemicals. Anthocyanins from berries and grapes also decrease UV-associated skin cancer risk and skin cell damage. Anthocyanins, and their related chemical cousins proanthocyanins from the seeds of grapes, prevent the breakdown of collagen and improve blood flow. In addition, when they are eaten, these chemicals have been shown in experimental studies to maintain the skin levels of a critically important antioxidant called glutathione.

TURMERIC

The South Asian spice turmeric, the ingredient that gives curry a distinctive dark orange-yellow color, contains an antioxidant called curcumin. In keeping with our theme, curcumin has major antioxidant and anti-inflammatory properties.

Turmeric has a long history of use in India as a medicinal agent for skin diseases. Recent studies in psoriasis, scleroderma, and wound healing have all supported the notion that the antioxidant and anti-inflammatory properties of curcumin extend into the skin. With regard to anti-aging properties, curcumin, which makes up about 3 percent of turmeric, has been shown to lower the risk of UV-induced cancer in a number of experimental studies. It has also been shown to enhance collagen production and the manufacture of glycosaminoglycans.

While we need more human studies on skin conditions, oral administration of curcumin does appear to have a significant anti-inflammatory influence in the joints and other human tissue far removed from the gastrointestinal tract. At the time of this writing, several pharmaceutical companies were developing topical curcumin preparations, including a gel delivery format for the reduction of inflammation in the skin.

GINGER

Since turmeric and ginger are in the same plant family, it shouldn't be too surprising that ginger would have similar anti-inflammatory and antioxidant properties. Ginger shares a similar story with a very long history of recorded medicinal use throughout Asia. Orally consumed ginger exerts significant anti-inflammatory activity, strong enough to provide relief in osteoarthritis patients. The anti-inflammatory chemicals in ginger also provide protection against UV exposure for the skin.

One unique characteristic of ginger is that, according to research published in the journal *Pharmacology and Therapeutics* (2006), it prevents the breakdown of elastin and the otherwise inevitable formation of wrinkles in experimental animals exposed to UV radiation. Both ginger and turmeric can be consumed in curries or incorporated into meals ranging from steamed vegetables to fish dishes. Since both turmeric and ginger can put the brakes on collagen-busting, skin age-inducing PGE2, they would be a top choice for the maintenance of healthy, youthful skin.

SESAME AND SEAWEED

Sesame seeds contain antioxidant chemicals that can help to protect the fats that make up our cell walls. The seeds contain a fibrous component called sesame lignans that has been shown to lower bad (LDL) cholesterol; help to enhance the antioxidant activity of vitamin E; and preserve important omega-3 fatty acid levels. Black sesame seeds contain significantly more antioxidants within their colorful fiber and may go even further in protecting cells against free-radical damage. Black sesame seeds and ground black-sesame paste for entrees, baked goods, and smoothies are available at Asian grocery stores.

Seaweeds are another highly nutritious food and a great source of antioxidants. New experimental research shows that seaweeds can protect skin cells against UV damage. The longest living people in the world, the Japanese, frequently consume sesame and seaweeds.

HONORABLE MENTIONS

Plenty of other foods can help reduce inflammation and provide a significant antioxidant boost. Whole grains, for example, are best known for keeping blood sugar balanced, enhancing satiety, and improving bowel function. Whole grains also carry significant antioxidants in the fibrous portion of the cereal. Oat bran and granola cereals have impressive antioxidant properties.

BRAN AND YOUR DERMIS

A study in the *Journal of Medicinal Foods* (2008) showed that the bran from Indian sorghum can inhibit the enzyme that breaks down our GAGs. Recall that the GAGs are the structural components of the dermis and provide overall volume to the skin. Specifically, the sorghum bran put the brakes on the enzyme that attacks our important hyaluronic acid, the major GAG component in the dermis.

Nuts, especially walnuts (which are very rich in omega-3), pecans, and hazelnuts have very high antioxidant properties. Walnuts provide eight times more antioxidant protection per gram than peanuts and even double that of the much-heralded blueberry.

Then we have the culinary spices. We have already mentioned ginger and turmeric, but let's not forget cinnamon, cloves, oregano, and parsley. All of these minor dietary items could easily be overlooked in fast-food-driven dietary choices. Turns out that cinnamon provides thirty times the antioxidant protection per gram of blueberries—and cloves provide even more protection! Keep culinary herbs and spices in full view to remind you of their necessity. Your skin will thank you for it.

DIETARY SUPPLEMENTS

Most of the dietary items discussed in this chapter have both antioxidant and anti-inflammatory activity. This provides a protective double-edge because oxidative stress and free radicals cause inflammation in the skin, and, in turn, inflammatory chemicals promote further oxidative stress and free-radical generation. Obviously, dietary agents that can halt this cycle of skin damage would be good candidates for inclusion in skin-healthy dietary supplements.

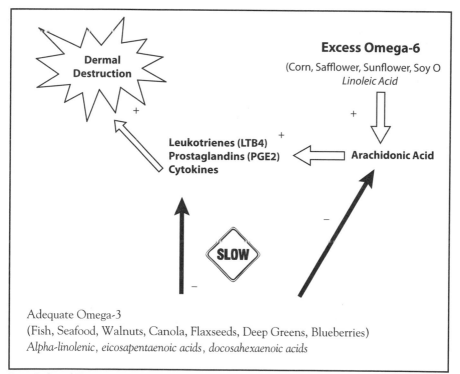

Diet-Induced Destruction: Excess omega-6-rich oils promote (+) the production of three classes of inflammatory chemicals (PGE2, LTB4, and cytokines) that destroy the dermal structures and skin's barrier function. Omega-3 fatty acids can help inhibit (–) the production of these inflammatory chemicals.

3

Sugar and the AGEing Skin

> "*Certain features of the American diet are, we believe, of significance in dermatological management. Americans consume excessive quantities of carbohydrate as compared to other populations of the world. Accordingly, diets involving a reduction in carbohydrate assume greater importance in American than in European dermatology.*"

THE AUTHORS OF THIS 1942 QUOTE from the textbook *Fundamentals of Medical Dermatology* were specifically referring to excessive carbohydrates as including dietary sugar and its role in the promotion of inflammatory skin conditions. Almost seventy years ago, these dermatologists were naming names among the carbohydrates, calling out fountain drinks, juices, ice cream, white flour products, puffed cereal grains, bar candies, and, as they called them, fountain delicacies.

They went on to lay out a protocol for sugar reduction, advice that we personally find a great modern-day template for healthy eating. Specifically, they recommended consuming whole wheat bread, whole grain bran-containing cereals without added sugar, potatoes baked with jackets, whole fruits only (not juices), two or more green vegetables at a meal, and a minimum of three vegetables and a salad every day. Pasta and rice were to be limited. This is timeless advice for healthy skin and the limitation of the skin-aging process.

Whatever attraction North Americans may have had in 1942 to added sugars has now become, as outlined in chapter 1, a full-blown love affair. Our inability to resist the sweet temptress is reflected by the fact that added sugar—that specifically and purposefully added into foods and beverages— accounts for more than 30 percent of all carbohydrates consumed. Approximately half of all added sugar is in the form of cheap and intensely sweet high-fructose corn syrup (HFCS).

HFCS has moved rapidly into our food supply since the early 1970s, making its way into baked goods, beverages, dairy products, desserts, candies, canned fruits, and jellies—and mirroring the rise in obesity. HFCS is the technologically inspired joining of two of the simplest sugars—fructose and glucose. Some researchers consider HFCS to be different, and potentially more health compromising, than even white table sugar (sucrose), which also contains glucose and fructose.

Whether this is true or not remains to be seen. However, the real concern is that both sucrose and HFCS consumption ultimately carry lots and lots of glucose and fructose into our bloodstream and onwards to our skin. Once there, glucose and particularly fructose will wreak havoc to skin structures. Inside the dermis, there is a wicked attraction between these sugars and the proteins in our collagen. The end result is always bad for collagen, which has its structure twisted and contorted by a process called cross-linking.

Skin Sugar

Dermatologist Erich Urbach, MD, was the first to show that a diet high in sugar can not only influence blood sugar, but also significantly elevate skin sugar levels. He used biopsies of skin and reported in the *Archives of Dermatology and Syphilology* (1945) that a low-sugar diet was associated with far less sugar within the skin of adults. As if we needed any more reasons to take in fish oil, he showed that the addition of cod-liver oil to the standard diet could lower skin sugar levels. In fact, the fasting skin sugar levels of animals fed cod-liver oil for just one week were 23 percent lower, even with no appreciable difference in blood-sugar levels.

Obviously preventing elevations in skin sugar levels is a good thing. Excess sugar hanging around the skin layers will only promote inflammation and oxidative stress. One finding buried in the study was largely dismissed, but it would turn out to be a gold nugget of information pertaining to skin aging.

These researchers reported that the sugar in the skin wasn't completely free sugar in glucose form. Rather, a large percentage of it was joined to proteins—*sucre proteidique* (sugar protein), as they referred to it in honor of the French researcher who coined the term. They also reported that those with a history of continually high blood-sugar levels had far higher levels of sugar bound up to proteins in the skin.

The significance of these findings was enormous, although not appreciated at the time. It would be decades before dietary sugars bonding with proteins were proven to cause malformations of collagen and elastin in the dermis. The process would come to be called glycation of dermal structures, and it is a central factor in aging your skin.

The Sugar-Glycation Process

Collagen and elastin are the scaffolding and structural cage of the skin. Individual units of collagen are linked together with other fibers by a very organized set of cross-links. Each long rope-like strand of collagen is joined together by smaller ropes at evenly spaced, specific locations. The end result is a large net with much greater stability and tensile strength than individual ropes alone. The same purposeful cross-linking of individual elastin fibers to one another also provides strength and stability to the elastin network. Nature set it up perfectly; the cross-links provide just the right amount of strength and stability, yet are not too strong and stiff because excessive cross-linking would take away from the elasticity and flexibility of our skin.

Natural cross-links in the normal dermal matrix do not involve sugar. An entirely different set of inappropriate cross-linking occurs when excess sugar arrives like a gate-crasher in the dermis. Glucose and fructose catch the eye of the amino acids of collagen and elastin. They join together in a covalent bonding process called glycation, and after some dehydrating and rearranging here and there, the pair come to be known as an Advanced Glycation End-product, with an acronym that couldn't be any more appropriate—AGE.

The AGE clinging to the collagen is called an adduct. As time passes, the adduct team gets bored and reaches out for another amino acid to form a separate collagen rope, resulting in excess cross-linking. The collagen and elastin fibers are now joined together in locations that are not part of the natural and beneficial cross-linking process. The consequence, as you might imagine, is the loss of the youthful elasticity of the skin. To make matters worse, the AGE is much more likely to cross-link with other collagen fibers after UV exposure and in the presence of excess free radicals.

Researchers writing in the *British Journal of Dermatology* (2001) reported that the glycation process in the skin is turned on in earnest at age thirty-five, with progressive increases in AGE content thereafter. This supports the findings of Italian researchers who reported almost two decades ago that glycation in our dermal collagen gets fired up when we reach our late twenties, after which glycated collagen will accumulate in the dermis at a rate of 3.7 percent per year. Over a decade, that can add up quickly, and the actual percentage is highly dependent upon diet and lifestyle choices.

Once initiated, the glycation process can actually inactivate certain antioxidant enzymes, including the UV- and collagen-protecting antioxidant enzymes that play important defensive roles. Incredibly, the AGEs are not satisfied with cross-linking our collagen and elastin. They also appear to cross-link these important antioxidant enzymes at their own amino acid joints, rendering them useless!

Unlike the epidermis, which turns over or replicates in a month or less, collagen fibers are relatively long-lasting structures. While it can take years to fully replace collagen fibers, there is an ongoing process of repair, demolition, and reconstruction in the dermis. Normally spaced collagen nets, those with proper cross-linking, allow room for the repair processes to occur. A massive problem occurs, however, when extra sugar-induced collagen cross-links are in place. Tightly bound collagen ropes in unnatural formation are separated only by a tiny molecule of sugar, and this impedes the ability of the larger repair enzymes to get in and fix the problem. The repair enzymes want nothing more than to get to work and break those sugar bonds, but they can't squeeze in the narrow space to get the job done right.

This problem is compounded by the fact that some of the repair processes are performed to only some degree, leaving a half-finished job. It's like taking apart an appliance and then realizing that you only have a large screwdriver to repair a microprocessor. The end result is that the repairing and replacing of collagen takes far longer, leaving even more time for sugar and collagen proteins to produce further cross-linking. While some degree of excess cross-linking is an inevitable part of the aging process, it is a vicious circle that is undoubtedly fueled by excess dietary sugars.

To see firsthand the influence of consistently high sugar delivery to the skin, we need only look to diabetes. Patients with diabetes are much more likely to have high levels of sugars bound to proteins in the skin. Diabetes accelerates the development of AGE-altered collagen. If elevated sugar delivery to the skin is indeed a central issue in aging the skin, then balancing blood sugar and insulin would help keep AGE collagen destruction in check.

In a now classic study in the *Journal of Clinical Investigation* (1991), researchers from Belfast, Northern Ireland, showed that improving glycemic control can significantly decrease the glycation of skin collagen. Using skin biopsies, they showed that simply providing advice on how to properly check blood sugar with a home device can decrease glycated collagen formation by 25 percent over just four months. It is important to emphasize prevention, because once AGE-induced cumulative damage occurs to collagen, it is resistant to reversal.

The inhibition of AGE formation through diet and select supplements is the key to preventing unwanted collagen cross-linking. Since excess dietary glucose and fructose can accelerate the accumulation of AGE-altered collagen in the skin, it would be logical to think that a very low carbohydrate and high protein diet would be the key to keeping skin AGEing in check. Yet when researchers from Dartmouth Medical School placed adults on an Atkins-style high-protein diet for two to four weeks, they actually found increases in AGE formation. One particular AGE, known to be a big-time collagen cross-linker, doubled during the minimal carbohydrate diet!

> Whole grains, fruits, and vegetables are considered carbohydrates on the Atkins diet. Avoidance of these carbohydrates increased AGE. This means that all carbohydrates cannot be painted with the same brush. It also means that adhering to fad diets without plant-based antioxidants is the equivalent of applying a daily self-wrinkling cream.

The whole grains, fruits, and vegetables avoided on Atkins-style diets are not the major culprits in spiking blood sugar. Furthermore, avoidance of these foods means avoidance of antioxidants and anti-inflammatory nutrients. Certain foods and culinary herbs actually contain AGE-inhibiting chemicals. The Atkins diet also stimulates AGE production for another reason—the cooking techniques used to make these high-protein foods. As it turns out, we not only make AGEs in the skin when sugars and proteins unite, we also can deliver them preformed directly to the skin via the foods and beverages we consume.

Dietary AGE

The knowledge that AGEs are found in cooked foods containing sugars and amino acids is not new. We have known that heat can form AGEs for a century. The reaction changes the food, quite often enhancing its color, aroma, and flavor. We are lured by the seductive taste of AGE-rich foods. Sometimes we can even see the formation of AGEs when foods turn brown, such as on the outer crust of bread or oven-roasted poultry skin. However, just because a dietary item doesn't have a distinctive dark-brown coat, it does not mean the item is AGE-free.

When it comes to AGE formation in food, moisture matters. Foods prepared with high heat in the absence of water—such as oven-roasted, grilled, or fried meats—are AGE heavyweights. Much lower AGEs are found in foods prepared in the presence of moisture by boiling, poaching, stewing, or steaming. This is regardless of whether the food is largely protein-rich or carbohydrate-rich. Consider these nutrition facts:

- Crispy rice cereal contains 220 times more AGEs per gram than boiled rice.
- Fast-food fries contain 87 times more AGEs per gram than a boiled spud.
- A fried egg has 62 times more AGEs than a poached egg.
- A serving of oven-fried and breaded Atlantic whiting has 16 times more dietary AGEs per gram than salmon sushi.
- Biscotti has 30 times more AGEs per gram than a toasted bagel.

The bottom line is that foods cooked for extended periods with so-called high and dry heat—at high temperatures with no moisture—are the foods most likely to be massive contributors to your AGE load and your skin AGEing.

Low oral consumption of dietary AGEs prevents inflammation and oxidative stress. Higher dietary AGE consumption is consistently associated with higher blood markers of inflammation.

Even when total calorie content is kept equal, a low-AGE diet can reduce blood levels of AGEs by 30 percent after just three days. Since higher blood levels of AGEs are associated with greater inflammation and oxidative stress, a 30 percent reduction in circulating AGEs is significant for your collagen and elastin.

Even a single high-AGE beverage has been shown to impair blood flow in patients with diabetes. This was observed after only ninety minutes of AGE consumption and lasted, in some cases, for as long as six hours. As we go through the aging process, our ability to eliminate food-based AGEs via the kidneys will decline. For this reason, it is even more important for older adults to stew, steam, poach, and boil foods.

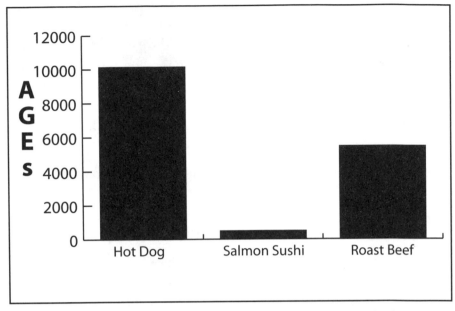

AGEs in kilounits (kU) per serving: Broiled hot dog, raw salmon, and roast beef. (Goldberg, et al. *Journal of the American Dietetic Association* 2004.)

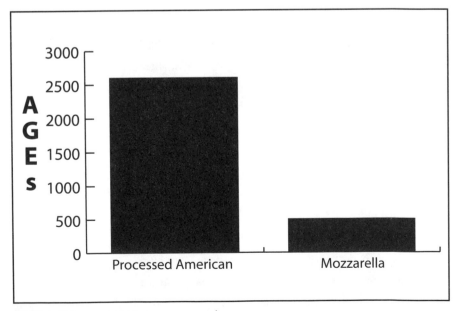

AGEs in kU per serving in two common cheeses.

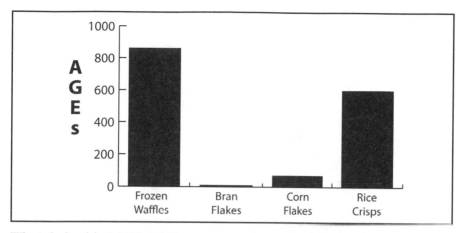

What's for breakfast? AGEs in kU per serving in four common breakfast options.

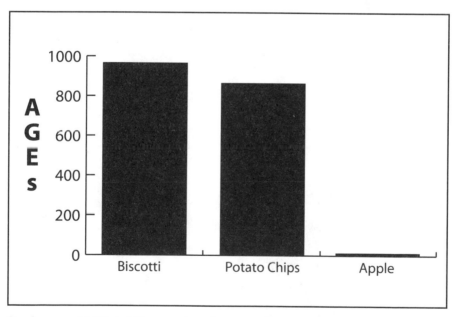

Snack anyone? AGEs in kU per serving of some snack options.

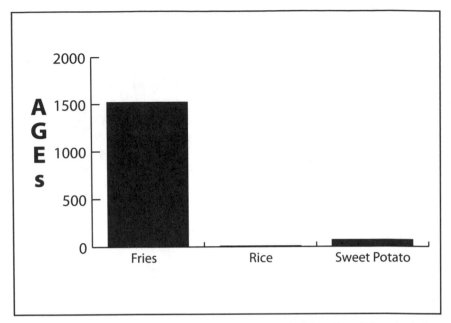

How about a side of…? AGEs in kU per serving of some side dishes. French fries, boiled rice, or a roasted sweet potato.

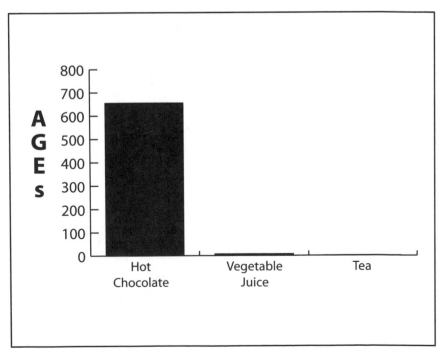

Caution! The beverage you are about to enjoy may AGE your skin: mass-marketed hot "cocoa" provides minimal antioxidants, lots of fat, sugar, and a whole lot of AGEs in kU per cup.

We cannot overstate the importance of reducing dietary AGEs in the maintenance of youthful skin and the prevention of visible signs of aging. We are estimated to consume about 75 milligrams of AGEs per day in our diet, and other chemicals that are closely related to and easily converted to AGEs may exceed 1,000 milligrams per day. Now we ask you, would you ever take a 1,000-milligram supplement of anything that may wrinkle your skin? Of course not. Yet decisions to cook and consume foods prepared with high and dry heat are in essence like taking that wrinkling tablet every day. Think about that the next time biscotti are passed around at the office party.

Yet another negative effect of higher dietary AGE consumption is that it is associated with an increased elimination of zinc from the body. Zinc plays an important antioxidant and anti-inflammatory role in the skin and has been shown to help acne as a supplement, so enhanced elimination of zinc via the urine would hardly be good for the skin.

AGE-Inhibitors

Now that we have covered the mechanisms behind sugar-induced and direct dietary AGE-induced cross-linking, let's delve into other ways to combat glycation—besides obviously keeping sugar intake and dietary AGEs low. Since AGEing of the skin is ratcheted up in the presence of high states of oxidative stress in the skin, antioxidants play a role in the prevention of skin AGEing. The good news is that scientists have been examining ways to prevent glycation with increased intensity and have uncovered some simple nutrient-based interventions to put the brakes on the process.

While agents that actually break up AGEs and undo the disastrous damage of cross-links remain the Rosetta stone of skin-aging research, AGE formation can be inhibited and prevented. Many of the dietary items discussed in the last chapter, those with potent antioxidant and anti-inflammatory activity, have also been shown to possess AGE-inhibiting properties. For example:

- Star culinary herb turmeric, or more specifically its curcumin, has been shown to reduce glycation and cross-linking of dermal collagen in diabetic animals.

- French researchers have shown that blueberry extract can reduce AGE products in the dermis and turn off MMP enzymes that would otherwise destroy collagen.
- Canadian researchers have shown that antioxidant chemicals within the blueberry plant, even in the leaves and stems, have anti-AGE activity.
- A team from India reported that oral green tea can reduce AGE formation and prevent collagen cross-linking in animals with consistently high blood sugar.
- Japanese researchers have shown that lycopene-rich tomato paste can prevent AGE formation.

Here are some other natural agents with AGE-inhibiting properties:

CINNAMON

An ideal candidate for AGE inhibition would be one with strong antioxidant activity and the ability to balance blood sugar. Cinnamon pocesses both of these fine qualities. Oral cinnamon extract enhances the repair and regeneration of damaged collagen. One of the naturally occurring chemicals in cinnamon has recently been identified as an active factor in the regulation of blood sugar. In fact, 1 to 3 grams of cinnamon extract is helpful in blood-sugar regulation among adults with type 2 diabetes.

Like many culinary spices, cinnamon is loaded with antioxidants, and a number of these chemicals are AGE-inhibitors. The Atkins diet may be able to generate a glycation product known to cross-link collagen, but cinnamon can trap this fat cat of glycation and inactivate it. You can think of cinnamon as a true bodyguard, taking the bullet for you as the glycation molecule forms an adduct (union) with cinnamon before it can turn into a full-blown AGE and destroy your collagen. The interesting part is that the AGE-inhibiting properties of cinnamon are not solely attributed to the antioxidant activity. The structural ability of cinnamon chemicals to bind with glycation chemicals makes the difference.

> Researchers from the University of Georgia reported in 2008 that among two dozen herbs and spices, cinnamon, cloves, oregano, and allspice have potent glycation-inhibiting properties and are capable of protecting our proteins from fructose-induced AGE formation.

GINGER

Another antioxidant-rich culinary spice, ginger is near the top of the AGE-inhibiting list. According to a report in the *British Journal of Nutrition* (2008), ginger reduced sugar-protein AGE formation by an incredible 93 percent under experimental conditions. Under these testing conditions, cinnamon was still a very close second at 88 percent inhibition of AGE formation, followed by cumin, green tea, black pepper, and basil.

GARLIC

Best known as a heart-healthy herb, garlic has a long history of use in treating the diseases associated with human aging. Garlic has long been noted to contain important antioxidant phytochemicals. The latest study, published in the *European Journal of Pharmacology* (2007), shows that aged garlic extract can, much like cinnamon, throw its body onto the live grenade of AGE-promoting chemicals. Specifically, Japanese Kyolic aged garlic extract was shown to prevent protein fragmentation and AGE cross-linking. This AGE-inhibition is thought to be due to the high concentration of the natural chemical S-allyl cysteine in garlic. Note that aged garlic extract has fifty times more S-allyl cysteine than raw garlic. Aged garlic extract is also well known for turning on the UV-protecting and anti-skin-aging SOD antioxidant enzyme.

ALPHA-LIPOIC ACID

Known as the universal antioxidant because it works in both water-soluble and fat-soluble environments, alpha-lipoic acid (ALA) is one of our most potent defenders. As with cinnamon, ALA improves blood sugar control and may help to prevent the effects of heavy-metal toxicities. While the primary function of ALA is the manufacture of energy within the mitochondria of our cells, it also helps repair damaged proteins. Likely because of its own antioxidant activity, ALA has been shown to preserve and recycle our other antioxidants, including vitamins C and E.

In 2004, researchers from India showed that, as expected, fructose can significantly increase glycation, AGE formation, and collagen cross-linking in skin. They also noted a reduction in vitamin C levels with dietary fructose consumption. However, when animals received ALA at the same time, there was marked decreases in AGE formation and decreased damage to collagen despite the high fructose intake. The results have been replicated, and researchers reported in the journal *Pharmazie* (2005) that ALA has significant AGE-inhibiting properties in the presence of a high-sugar diet.

CARNITINE

Carnitine has a known ability to balance blood sugar and insulin. Like alpha-lipoic acid, carnitine also plays an important role in the energy packet inside our skin cells, the mitochondria. When mitochondrial function becomes sub-par, especially through the aging process, we feel less energetic, and our skin appearance suffers.

Dysfunctional mitochondria in our skin cells increases free-radical generation and steps up the aging process. But carnitine can significantly reduce the AGEing of dermal collagen. In the presence of a high-fructose diet, carnitine can preserve antioxidants, sequester glycation chemicals, and prevent collagen cross-linking in animals.

TAURINE

This sulfur-containing amino acid compound is rich in fish and seafood. Smaller amounts are found in meats, yet it is largely absent from the vegetarian diet. Some species of algae are the only option for taurine in the plant-based diet. Taurine helps to prevent damage to the lipid (fat) components of our cells. A number of animal studies show that taurine helps to prevent the free-radical damage normally induced by a diet high in sugar, and the amino acid's ability to help balance insulin and blood sugar was first noted in the 1930s.

In following with an obvious theme, taurine helps with the manufacture of energy and protects the mitochondria from the damage of aging and illness. Three separate studies in 2004 and 2005, including one in the *Journal of Diabetes and Its Complications* (2005), showed that taurine can prevent damage to collagen and AGE-induced cross-linking of dermal collagen when supplemented to animals on a high-fructose diet.

CARNOSINE

This small protein, or dipeptide, has well-known antioxidant activity and, like taurine, is found almost exclusively in animal meats. Carnosine helps regulate blood sugar and insulin. The first indication that carnosine has anti-glycation properties came more than fifteen years ago. Researchers from Australia showed that carnosine seems to offer itself up for glycation and, at the same time, protects important structures against damage. Over the years, many experimental studies have shown that carnosine can prevent AGE formation and limit destructive AGE-induced cross-linking. As mentioned earlier, AGEs try to knock out our important anti-skin-aging enzyme SOD, so it is comforting to know that carnosine can help protect SOD from AGE-induced cross-linking.

VEGETARIANS AND AGING SKIN

A plant-based diet offers many benefits. However, some careful considerations must be made to cover all skin-friendly, collagen-building nutrient bases while on a vegetarian diet. Recently, researchers reported in the *Annals of Nutrition and Metabolism* (2008) that vegetarian adults have lowered rates of collagen production. Unexpectedly, researchers have found that the blood levels of AGEs are much higher in long-term vegetarians than in those consuming a mixed plant-and-animal diet.

The AGE-inhibiting amino acids taurine and carnosine are mostly absent from the plant-based diet. Taurine is found in high concentration in fish and seafood, and both taurine and carnosine are found in animal meats. For vegetarians and vegans, this dietary deficiency may create a problem related to glycation.

Three reasons have been suggested for this unexpected finding among vegetarians—the first is the greater likelihood of heavy consumption of carbohydrates, and fructose in particular, from high fruit intake. Fructose overload is certainly plausible since vegetarians have been shown to consume twice as much fruit as omnivores. The second is the greater reliance upon dairy products. (In one study, vegetarians reported double the dairy consumption versus non-vegetarians.) As discussed earlier, some dairy products can be rich in preformed AGEs.

Finally, a meat-, fish-, and seafood-free diet is devoid of taurine, carnosine, and omega-3 EPA intake. Since all three of these nutrients can prevent AGE formation, it has been theorized that the deficiency might be at play. Supplementation with a vegan protein with concentrated taurine and carnosine may be advised.

FLAVONOIDS

Some members of the flavonoid family of phytochemicals have been shown to put the brakes on AGE formation in experimental settings. Luteolin is a flavonoid found in artichoke leaves, celery, green peppers, and green leafy herbs such as parsley, thyme, and mint. Luteolin is a potent AGE inhibitor, reducing glycation by 78 percent. Its naturally occurring chemical cousins, quercetin and rutin, also have AGE-inhibiting properties. Quercetin is found in high amounts in red onions, tea, apples, grapes, berries, and green leafy vegetables, and inhibits glycation by 65 percent. Rutin is found in high amounts in apples, citrus fruits, cherries, prunes, and rose hips, and inhibits glycation by 69 percent.

BENFOTIAMINE

We have saved the best stand-alone AGE inhibitor for last. This is the fat-soluble form of thiamine, or vitamin B_1. It is much more readily absorbed and more effective at actually getting to the tissue to do its good deeds than synthetic thiamine is. Benfotiamine inhibits AGE formation. One of the reasons that benfotiamine is the reigning heavyweight AGE-inhibiting champion, the agent we have the most confidence in for AGE-inhibition in your skin, lies in the fact that its abilities are supported by human studies. The other nutrients and supplement ingredients discussed to this point will almost certainly work in synergistic fashion to stop AGEing skin in humans. For now, however, benfotiamine stands alone as the single product of choice.

The first human study, published in the journal *Diabetes* (2000), showed that taking 600 milligrams of benfotiamine for twenty-eight days significantly reduces AGE formation. One of the most potent chemicals of glycation, the infamous cross-linking producer called methylglyoxal, was inhibited by almost 70 percent. The second human study, published more recently in *Diabetes Care* (2006), showed that the co-administration of benfotiamine with a high-AGE meal can limit the otherwise expected rise in blood levels of AGE and prevent blood-flow abnormalities.

Oral administration of benfotiamine appears to have both acute and long-term benefits. As we go to press, researchers are perfecting topical benfotiamine applications to limit skin aging. Supplemental vitamin B_6 along with benfotiamine may provide additional efficacy, since research shows that B_6 can limit the production of protein-sugar chemicals that can otherwise be modified easily to form AGEs.

Skin AGE Content as a Mirror of Health

You know now that a wrinkle is not just a wrinkle. The visual signs of aging are, in fact, a reflection of internal health. Looking older than one's age is associated with heart, lung, and kidney diseases—and these are only the conditions that have actually been investigated. Since looking old for one's age is associated with an increased risk of mortality, or dying earlier, other chronic medical conditions also are almost certainly associated with an increased risk of the visible signs of aging. The AGE story provides even more proof of this concept.

Blood and skin levels of AGEs have been linked to age-related diseases for a number of years. In chapter 1, for example, we said that diminished kidney filtration is associated with looking old for one's age and more visible wrinkles. Interestingly, the kidney is a primary route of AGE elimination from the body, and any slowdown in filtration will give more AGEs an extended opportunity to do damage. Skin AGE levels also correlate with kidney function, and higher skin AGEs, as you would imagine, are associated with decreased kidney function.

Until recently, skin measurements for AGE content were performed by use of biopsy. A new area of investigation is the use of a noninvasive AGE reader developed by European scientists. In 1997, researchers from the Netherlands serendipitously discovered that skin AGEs can be measured through light reflected back from the skin. With the AGE Reader, illuminating light enters the skin and the amount of AGEs present in the skin layers influence the absorption of light.

Over the last decade, researchers have shown that the AGE Reader is a reliable way to measure overall risk of cardiovascular disease, kidney disease, and, of course, diabetic complications. Again, one need not actually have diabetes to see an association with high skin-AGE content and internal ill-health via the AGE Reader assessment. The reliability and simplicity of the device's use have driven dermatologists' interest, and the AGE Reader is destined for North American dermatology offices.

The higher the skin AGE content, the more likely you are to have fragmented collagen, disturbed elastin, and a weak dermal structure. The higher your skin AGE content, the higher your oxidative stress and inflammation burden, and obviously, the more likely you will be to have a wrinkled appearance. Finally, the higher the skin AGE content, the more likely you will be to have an early progression of age-related diseases—heart, kidney, lung, brain, and other—initiated in the body.

A new study in the journal *Experimental Gerontology* (2008) is quite alarming because it showed much higher skin AGE levels among overweight young people. This connection was not without consequence because overweight adults less than forty years old were also more likely to have impaired skin elasticity based on objective testing. This does not bode well for the future: Spanish researchers have also shown that young adults are most likely to be drawn to a high-preformed AGE diet via fast and convenient foods.

Worse still is a 2008 ComPsych study showing that only 18 percent of corporate workers in their thirties had a diet consisting of healthy foods and only 20 percent were exercising on a regular basis. Combined with UV exposure and EMF from the wireless world, this creates the perfect storm for a new generation with AGE-induced wrinkle enhancement.

Dietary AGEs and the Gut Bacteria

The human gastrointestinal tract (GI) is home to more than five hundred species of bacteria. The good guys in this bunch, the beneficial bacteria, are unsung heroes in the promotion of our health. Collectively, the gut bacteria is referred to as our intestinal microflora. A healthy microflora is essential to AGE detoxification. *Lactobacillus* and *Bifidobacteria* are two essential species that help make up a healthy microflora. Both have been associated with health and longevity. These bacteria are found in great numbers within fermented foods and yogurts.

Again, the North American situation is not good when it comes to the intestinal microflora: many people are experiencing a diet-induced loss of health-promoting *Lactobacillus* and *Bifidobacteria* strains. This pertains to AGE because these so-called friendly bacteria are essential for the absorption of many of the antioxidants and nutrient AGE-inhibitors previously described. The good bacteria release AGE-inhibiting chemicals from plant foods that arrive in the intestines. Indeed, experimental studies show that bacteria from a healthy microflora can help to eliminate AGEs.

The AGEs, however, are not content to sit by idly and watch themselves be dominated by *Lactobacillus* and *Bifidobacteria*. Dietary AGEs can diminish the levels of good bacteria. Dietary glycation products, sugar linked to proteins, have specific anti-bacterial activity against *Bifidobacteria* and promote the growth of undesirable gut bacteria associated with inflammation and cancer. This influence of dietary AGEs on *Bifidobacteria* is most pronounced in the presence of disturbed intestinal microflora. In other words, if you have an abnormal gut-bacterial profile up front, and according to some researchers, that means seven of every ten adults, dietary AGEs will make a bad situation worse by further diminishing levels of good bacteria.

Again, having low levels of the good bacteria means fewer AGE-inhibiting chemicals absorbed for your protection. We will discuss the importance of a healthy gut microflora for youthful, glowing skin in more detail next chapter. For now, it represents just one more reason to keep dietary AGE in check.

The Skin AGE Reduction Plan

At this point, it should be very clear that glycation is the scourge of youthful skin and a major promoter of internal ill-health. Our nutritional plan and recipes to make your skin younger will place great priority on reducing consumption of foods containing preformed AGEs, while at the same time maximizing the intake of AGE-inhibiting foods and beverages.

> Avoid processed carbohydrates, processed sugars, and too much fructose. In protecting our collagen from the ravages of glycation, we must reduce the supply of raw materials, such as glucose and fructose, to a minimum. Any foods and beverages that spike blood sugar and insulin—and what processed carbohydrate, sugar-laden fountain delicacy doesn't?—are the enemy of collagen and elastin.

After making every effort to keep sugars to a bare minimum, the next step is to restrict preformed AGEs in our diets as an essential part of maintaining youthful, glowing skin. Massive reductions in the daily delivery of AGEs to the skin and reductions in oxidative stress and inflammation can be obtained by boiling, stewing, steaming, and poaching foods, or eating raw, uncooked greens in the form of salads. Even a moderate intake of preformed dietary AGEs will increase AGE delivery to the skin by some 10 percent in healthy adults.

Once you consume a grilled, fried, oven-roasted, or baked food prepared with high heat, you have transported yourself into the high skin–AGE bracket. It takes time and conditioning to steer clear of foods prepared with high and dry heat. In our recipe section in chapter 8, we have focused exclusively on steaming, soups, and salads as a reminder to keep moisture and lower temperatures as priorities. These foods carry lots of the antioxidants, AGE-inhibiting chemicals, and anti-inflammatory omega-3 fatty acids that we have discussed.

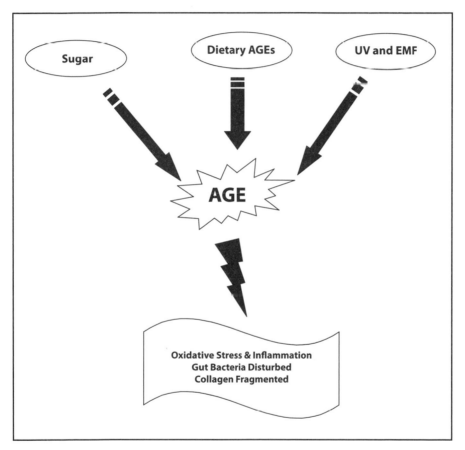

The AGE Explosion: Combine lots of dietary sugar and preformed dietary AGEs via foods cooked on high and dry heat. Throw in some ultraviolet rays and some electromagnetic exposure, and you have the recipe for dermal disaster. The skin-aging process goes into overdrive!

4

Skin Digestion:
The Gut-Skin Connection

> *"Everything has been thought of before. But the difficulty is to think of it again."—Goethe*

A S DISCUSSED IN CHAPTER 3, IMPORTANT intestinal bacteria can promote health and inhibit AGE. As soon as we take our first breath at birth, the once sterile environment of our gastrointestinal tract (GI) becomes home to legions of bacteria. As life goes on, more and more bacteria will set up camp in the intestines until you have about 10^{14} bacteria belonging to more than five hundred different species. The overwhelming majority of these bacteria reside in the large intestine, with relatively few bacteria in the stomach and small intestine. The normal intestinal bacteria are collectively referred to as microflora or just simply flora—and twenty-four hours a day, seven days a week, with no holidays or personal days off, they defend your health.

Among the many genera of bacteria that reside in the GI tract, two have a well-deserved reputation for promoting health. *Lactobacilli* and *Bifidobacteria* are the so-called friendly bacteria that you might recognize from yogurt labels. These two are involved in vitamin synthesis, detoxification and metabolism of toxic substances, stimulation of the immune response, and protection from pathogenic (bad) bacteria. Healthy intestinal microflora also create a barrier, a film-like coating over the inner lining of the intestinal wall. This film keeps toxins and bad bacteria from gaining access through the wall and into your bloodstream.

It may seem implausible that some bacterial residents of the gut might slow the skin-aging process. How could two distant bodily systems have such a relevant connection in the aging process—and what on earth do bacteria have to do with it? In addition to anti-glycation properties, we will provide many examples of how good bacteria can influence skin health. We have lots of information to cover. However, for perspective, we must step back in time to look at the scientific beginnings of the gut-skin connection. As we will see, a whole lot of the gut-and-skin aging connection was laid out for us more than a century ago.

Autointoxication Revisited

In 1901, William A. Lane, MD, of London was arguably the most famous surgeon in the world. He was called upon by the United Kingdom's upper crust, the rich and famous society folks, politicians, and Royals to perform his surgical trade. If reality TV had existed then, Lane would have been featured regularly on *Entertainment Tonight*. He, along with others in the late 1800s, was convinced that imperfect digestion, the decomposition of proteins and other food-based waste sitting in the colon, was a central issue in the development of human disease. Doctors and scientists of that era suspected that toxins from the gut were gaining access to the bloodstream and causing internal damage. When constipation and digestive dysfunction became a chronic issue, autointoxication was the toxic end result.

The term *intestinal autointoxication* refers to the notion that some diseases can arise from toxins produced within the gastrointestinal tract. While the name was new, the idea that the constipated colon was a source of toxicity was hardly a new concept. Even the ancient Egyptians suggested that toxic agents associated with feces were related to disease. The difference was that with the advancement of science, researchers in the late nineteenth century found that the decomposition of proteins in the intestines (termed *putrefaction*) could produce nasty chemicals that had the potential to cause illness.

For Lane, the absorption of toxins from the gut was the great promoter of the aging process—including the skin-aging process. He and another physician pal, Adolphe Combe, both stated that the skin became thin, without tone (uneven color), relaxed, inelastic, and wrinkled at an earlier age when things were consistently not running smoothly through the intestinal tract. Thinking as a surgeon, Lane figured why not just cut out the colon? And so in 1901 the anti-aging specialist performed the first of hundreds of surgeries, short-circuits as they were known, in which he cut out the colon. This was a completely absurd thing to do, and some patients lost lives in the process, yet the practice continued for more than a decade.

Perhaps there was a kinder, gentler way to address intestinal autointoxication and promote health through the aging process. Maybe we didn't need to literally cut our guts out to slow the inevitable aging process. Elie Metchnikoff, PhD, winner of the Nobel Prize in Medicine in 1908, also suggested that premature aging was related to toxins from the gut. However, his solution was not to cut out the colon. Instead, he took a more rational approach and advocated for altering the intestinal microflora.

Metchnikoff, who worked in the world-famous Pasteur Institute, claimed that not all the bacteria residing and passing through the gut were out to harm us, and he started to identify good bacteria and bad bacteria within the gut. In his 1907 book, *The Prolongation of Life*, Metchnikoff stated that some intestinal bacteria produce useful substances that may protect against premature aging. It was a novel concept and one that excited the public. Before the days of highly paid publicists, Metchnikoff garnered a two-page spread in the *New York Times Magazine* that covered his groundbreaking work. He theorized that harmful intestinal bacteria are responsible for the manufacture of toxins that shortened lifespan, but these harmful bacteria could be offset by good bacteria.

Among Europeans at that time, the Bulgarians, the Turks, and the Armenians had notable longevity. They were also reported to have fewer visible signs of aging despite advanced years. Commenting in his book on a woman of age 106, Metchnikoff noted that in contrast to expectations, "her skin was not extremely wrinkled." When he looked closely at the diets of all three European groups known for longevity, frequent consumption of fermented milk was the common thread. Specifically, two bacteria were identified in fermented milk, *Lactobacillus bulgaricus* and *Streptococcus thermophilus*. These were the first so-called good bacteria, soon joined by a third genera called *Bifidobacteria*. All three could inhibit the bacteria that were involved in putrefaction.

Metchnikoff recommended the good bacteria for skin diseases, which is interesting because it has been documented that Persian women used a fermented milk to "preserve the freshness of their complexions" centuries ago, long before *Lactobacillus bulgaricus* was identified. In any case, before long, *Lactobacillus bulgaricus* was into the hands of enthusiastic researchers, drug manufacturers, and milk companies who used it in oral and topical preparations.

The Dawn of the *Lactobacillus* Era

Some physicians gave anecdotal reports of the benefits of using *Lactobacillus bulgaricus* (or milk fermented with the bacteria) for skin conditions. However, the first formal scientific investigation was by European dermatologist Jaime Peyri, MD, who reported in the *Journal of Cutaneous Diseases* (1912) that topical *Lactobacillus bulgaricus* was helpful for acne and skin inflammation. At the time, researchers referred to this treatment as bacteriotherapy of the skin. Most of the products were made locally, some even by physicians themselves. The first major commercial oral *Lactobacillus* preparation went by the name Cultol (later revised to Neo-Cultol) and was brought to market in 1915. Cultol guaranteed doctors and consumers live, active bacteria for six months.

> Early probiotic preparations were marketed for their ability to provide glowing and vibrant health, as reflected through the appearance of the skin.

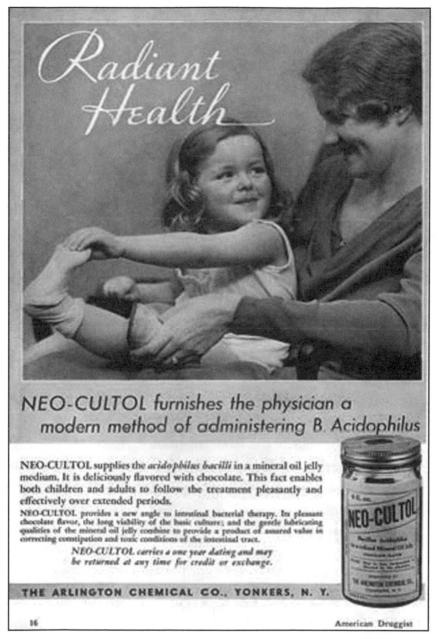

Lactobacillus acidophilus is advertised in the *American Druggist* magazine (1930).

Over time, more and more cases were published showing the value of oral *Lactobacillus* for general health. In the 1920s, researchers from Yale University and a separate group at the first meeting of the Canadian Dermatological Society both reported the benefit of oral *Lactobacillus acidophilus* in reducing skin inflammation. In the 1930s, oral *Lactobacillus* was reported helpful for a variety of skin conditions, acne and eczema in particular.

Respected Los Angeles dermatologist Moses Scholtz, MD, even endorsed a particular *Lactobacillus*-enhancing product called Lacto-Dextrin in the pages of the *California and Western Medicine* journal (1930). Lacto-Dextrin was a powdered formula described on the tin as "A Food for Changing the Intestinal Flora." Scholtz's general advice to dermatology patients in the 1930s, which we believe still holds true today, included staying away from excess sugars and proteins, choosing a broad diet "consisting chiefly of fruits and vegetables," and incorporating a fermented milk or *Lactobacillus* supplement into the action plan. No argument from us.

> *"It is not too much to say that one can foretell with considerable accuracy the intestinal flora of a person from his general appearance, and, above all, from the state of his skin."*
> —Dermatologist H.W. Barber, *British Medical Journal*, 1926

From the vantage point of the 1930s, these *Lactobacillus* products looked like they were here to stay. Generally, doctors seemed to like the results; consumers were on board; and credible manufacturers had entered in the arena. Then, just like the dinosaurs, the products vanished into thin air. A burgeoning industry seemed to disappear off the face of North America's consumer map within the blink of an eye.

Just like video killed the radio star, the discovery of antibacterial agents in 1935 forever changed the face of medicine and sealed the fate of Neo-Cultol and Lacto-Dextrin. Their old bottles and tins are now the stuff of flea markets and hunter-gatherers on eBay. By the late 1930s and early 1940s, the use of *Lactobacillus* by professionals had waned. The authors of the *Fundamentals of Medical Dermatology* stated in 1942, "Acidophilus therapy has fallen into disuse, but is of some value" in general dermatology. However, for the next two decades, the therapy was generally forgotten.

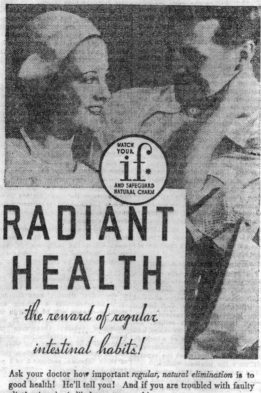

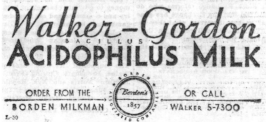

A *New York Times* (1932) ad for Borden's acidophilus milk infers that the probiotic beverage helps maintain radiant skin. Modern research is starting to back this up. (Used with permission by Hexion Specialty.)

Back to the Future Again!

Robert Siver, MD, a dermatologist from Baltimore, broke the silence in 1961 by performing an investigation using a new *Lactobacillus* product. An old-school doctor, he began using a *Lactobacillus* preparation called Lactinex in cases with marked gastrointestinal disturbances and then noticed a significant improvement in acne. This preparation, still on the market today, consists of two species of *Lactobacillus* bacteria: *Lactobacillus acidophilus* and *Lactobacillus bulgaricus*.

Now curious, Siver began to investigate the clinical value of *Lactobacillus* probiotics specifically for acne, even in the absence of overt gastrointestinal symptoms. Writing in the *Journal of the Medical Society of New Jersey* (1961), he reported the significant value of Lactinex among three hundred patients with acne. Siver states in the journal… "*Lactobacillus* is not a universal cure for acne…however, clinical experience suggests involvement of the metabolic products present in the preparation (Lactinex) and associated with the gastrointestinal tract. Interactions of skin manifestations of acne vulgaris and of metabolic processes of the intestinal tract are suggestive."

Around the same time, German dermatologist Gerhard Schmid-Ott, MD, PhD, was reporting great success with an oral *Bifidobacteria* strain in the treatment of eczema. These doctors were like lone wolves on each continent, but while the results were hardly far reaching in changing dermatological care, other rumblings were in the air. Groups in Japan and Russia followed by showing that applying *Lactobacillus* to the skin might confer protection against radiation.

Over time, it would become impossible to ignore these important bacteria and the links between the microbial residents of the GI tract and global aspects of health. In recent years, the good bacteria that reside in the gut have made a successful return to the international scientific spotlight, with research showing untold influences on areas far removed from the colon.

Some recent findings have implications for the maintenance of healthy, glowing skin. In 1999, a landmark study published in the prestigious British journal *Lancet* showed that orally administered probiotics to mothers during pregnancy and early lactation could decrease the risk of skin inflammation (eczema) in their infants. When the researchers followed up with the children four years later, they were still much less likely to experience eczema than the children of mothers who had taken only a placebo. Probiotics were back, and this time the science was being conducted on a firm foundation.

Exciting new research in the field of probiotics is not limited to the local effects of good intestinal bacteria on digestive disorders. Recently, bacteria belonging to these genera have been shown to lower the levels of inflammation-promoting and collagen-destroying immune chemicals called cytokines—not just locally in the gut, but also in the body-wide bloodstream when orally administered. The systemic anti-inflammatory effect of the oral probiotics is quite strong, capable of reducing joint inflammation in arthritic rats.

However, the research is not confined to animals. In human research published in the *American Journal of Clinical Nutrition* (2003), Swedish researchers showed that a strain of *Lactobacillus* had body-wide anti-inflammatory and antioxidant activity in smokers. The researchers showed a 37 percent reduction in blood markers of oxidative stress and a 42 percent reduction in blood levels of an inflammatory cytokine called IL-6.

Note that these are reductions of inflammatory chemicals beyond the gut. The findings have enormous implications for the long-term health of your skin. Keep in mind that IL-6 is an inflammatory chemical that is highly involved in the skin-aging process, and agents that keep IL-6 in check have been shown to have clinical benefit in reducing the visible signs of aging. The anti-aging skin ingredient Co-enzyme Q_{10}, for example, is known to inhibit IL-6 elevations as part of its action.

In support of the Swedish study, additional research also shows that species from the *Lactobacillus* and *Bifidobacteria* genera act as major antioxidants. Half a dozen studies have shown that probiotics protect against free radical damage and particularly against damage to the lipid (fat) component of cells. All of these studies underscore that the bacteria residing in the intestinal tract can have far-reaching effects, way beyond the gut.

A Porous Gut

Recall our discussion that normal intestinal bacteria spread a line of defense over the inner lining of the intestinal tract. This film prevents the passage of unwanted material through the gut lining and into body-wide circulation. In the 1980s and 1990s, researchers began to suspect that the overlap between skin and gut disturbances might be a result of a more porous intestinal lining. Studies in patients with inflammatory skin disorders showed that chemicals that should normally only remain on the internal, tube side of the GI tract were much more likely to pass through and enter the bloodstream and promote inflammation in the skin. When undesirable material passes into the blood, inflammatory chemicals will be unleashed. We contend that a porous or so-called leaky gut is also an issue in the acceleration of skin aging.

An eye-opening study in the journal *Digestive and Liver Disease* (2005) illustrates how improper bowel functioning can cause body-wide inflammation. Here, researchers found that chronic constipation is associated with significant changes in the intestinal microflora (with a lower level of beneficial *Lactobacillus* and *Bifidobacteria*) and a sharp increase in the permeability of the intestinal lining to undesirable material. The condition was also associated with an elevation in body-wide immune system activity. Chronic constipation provoked the manufacture of collagen-destroying inflammatory chemicals way beyond the local GI tract.

Increased permeability of the intestines is not only observed in constipation but also in irritable bowel syndrome, where there may be consistently loose stools. A more porous gut lining is also connected to small intestinal bacterial overgrowth (SIBO). When stomach acid becomes low due to aging or continuous use of antacid medications, bacteria can migrate upward from the colon and set up camp in the small intestine. The overgrowth can also occur when motility is limited in the GI tract—in other words, when things remain stagnant as in constipation.

Research published in the *Asia Pacific Journal of Clinical Nutrition* (2004) shows that a diet low in omega-3 fatty acids also encourages SIBO. A sedentary lifestyle and psychological stress can also compromise motility and cause a decrease in our good bacteria levels and an overgrowth of unwanted and unneeded bacteria in the small intestine. Symptoms of SIBO can include bloating, abdominal pain, constipation, diarrhea, gas, and even fatigue and pain distant from the intestinal sites.

The symptoms, especially the bloating, may be more evident soon after a meal high in carbohydrates and sugars because the bacteria in the small intestine have a field day fermenting the food. Basically, they turn your small intestine into a microbrewery of hydrogen and methane gas. Since our book is about youthful skin, we are more concerned with the reality that, due to bacterial interference in SIBO, proper absorption of proteins, fats, carbohydrates, B vitamins, and other nutrients becomes difficult.

THE DOWNSIDE OF ANTACIDS

Loss of stomach acid through the aging process and overprescription of stomach acid-blocking medications can set the stage for small intestinal bacterial overgrowth. Large numbers of bacteria can set up camp in the small intestine and successfully compete for nutrients that would otherwise be destined for your skin.

A recent study in *Clinical Gastroenterology and Hepatology* (2008) showed that SIBO is a significant factor in facial rosacea, even in younger adults. One thing is for sure: SIBO is much more likely to occur as we proceed through the aging process, and therefore, it is in our best interest to prevent its occurrence. *Lactobacillus* and *Bifidobacteria* supplements; fermented foods; omega-3-rich fish and seafood; lots of fiber-rich fruits, vegetables and whole grains; stress management; and exercise all can insulate against its occurrence.

Until about five years ago, most doctors and scientists laughed off autointoxication theories of illness and aging as nonsense. After all, many people with chronic constipation live healthy and normal lives into old age. Of course we could make the same argument about the proverbial chain smoker who dies peacefully while sleeping at ninety years old. Now, autointoxication has been resuscitated with updated research.

Autointoxication theorists appear to have been right in many regards one hundred years ago. Perhaps the cornerstone to youthful, radiant skin was, and still is, healthy intestinal microflora. As the research evolves, it is becoming clear that abnormal intestinal microflora is almost certainly driving increased intestinal permeability, or leaky gut, as it is called. We learned recently that *Lactobacillus* and *Bifidobacteria* secrete chemicals that help maintain the integrity of the gut lining. They also keep other bacteria in check, the undesirable sorts that produce enzymes that can otherwise break down the intestinal lining.

Bacteria within the intestinal tract can indeed influence the motility (or propulsion) of food and waste matter. Researchers have shown that *Lactobacilli* and *Bifidobacteria* actually normalize the passage of material through the intestines. Since the majority of North Americans have disturbances to the gut microflora, we contend that intestinal permeability, gut motility problems, and SIBO are a consideration not only for those with actual skin diseases but also for others. The occurrence of low-grade inflammation in the intestines, permeability of the gut lining, and overgrowth of bacteria in the small intestine are almost certainly more common than appreciated—undoubtedly the consistent influence of these factors will only add to the burden of inflammation and oxidative stress.

An Omega-3 Connection

Scientists have known since 1910 that a fiber-rich diet high in fruits, vegetables, and whole grains can promote the production of beneficial bacteria in the gut. On the other hand, a diet high in protein-rich animal foods (fermented dairy aside) in the absence of plant foods is associated with decreased *Lactobacillus* and *Bifidobacteria* in the gut. The reason is quite obvious: undigested fiber passes through the small intestine to the colon, where our friendly bacteria act upon it. The fiber is basically like a food for the health-protecting bacteria in our gut. Until recently a high-fat diet was considered to have a negative influence on the good bacteria. However, new research suggests that all fats are not alike in promoting or inhibiting the growth of our beneficial bacteria.

Consider research in the *Indian Journal of Gastroenterology* (2008) where fish oil was shown to be a growth promoter of *Bifidobacteria*, while beef fat decreases our good bacteria and increases the growth of bacteria associated with cancer. This is in line with other studies showing a dietary fat and intestinal-bacterial connection that seems more sophisticated than once imagined. Japanese researchers showed that among three different diets (one high in omega-6 corn oil, another high in beef fat, and a third high in fish oil), the fish oil group showed a beneficial effect on intestinal flora. Specifically, the fish-oil diet led to a threefold increase in *Bifidobacteria* and the lowest levels of the bacteria associated with cancer.

Additional experimental research has shown that a diet high in fish oil or flaxseed oil, both rich in omega-3, can increase *Lactobacilli*. Test-tube studies have shown that omega-6–rich corn oil and pure linoleic acid itself (the parent omega-6 oil) both inhibit the growth of *Bifidobacteria*. Pure EPA from fish oil, on the other hand, inhibits the potentially harmful and cancer-causing *Bacteroides* strains. Recall that dietary olive oil is linked to a decreased risk of the visible signs of aging, and it also appears to increase the growth of *Lactobacillus*.

Sophisticated research has shown that, in contrast to dietary saturated fats, polyunsaturated fats appear to influence the adhesion of good bacteria to our intestinal wall. Arachidonic acid, an inflammatory compound found in beef fat and manufactured from omega-6 vegetable oils (soybean, safflower, sunflower, and corn), causes less adhesion of good bacteria to intestinal cells. On the other hand, flaxseed oil, rich in omega-3, increases the adhesion of bacteria. Marine oils, high in EPA, have been shown to markedly increase the adhesion of *Lactobacillus* to the intestines.

Big in Japan

The Japanese diet contains elements that are known to positively influence intestinal microflora. Obviously there is a significant intake of omega-3 fatty acids from fish and seafood, lots of vegetables, and plenty of roots such as wasabi, daikon, and renkon. The three aforementioned roots are part of the *Brassica* family of vegetables, which have been shown to exert quite a specific growth of friendly bacteria in the human gut. The Japanese are known to be frequent consumers of *Brassica* family vegetables, and most often these are eaten with minimal cooking and have low AGE content.

Indeed, some specific items in the Japanese diet would normally escape consideration as promoters of good bacteria. For example, research shows that green tea promotes the growth of *Bifidobacteria*. How about all that fresh ginger that accompanies sushi? It has been reported that despite ginger's strong antimicrobial properties, it may actually contribute to the growth of *Lactobacilli*.

Honey is also a great way to sweeten foods because it contains antioxidant polyphenols, and at least two studies have shown that it can selectively promote the growth of *Bifidobacteria* and *Lactobacilli*. The dietary fiber, the omega-3 fatty acids from fish, the green tea, the *Brassicas*, and a host of other colorful phytonutrients within the Japanese diet may influence intestinal microflora in a beneficial way.

BRASSICA 101

The Brassica family of vegetables includes the following:

- Arugula
- Bok choy
- Broccoli
- Broccoli sprouts
- Broccolini
- Brussels sprouts
- Cabbage
- Cauliflower
- Chinese broccoli
- Daikon
- Horseradish
- Kale
- Kohlrabi
- Mustard greens
- Purple cauliflower
- Radish
- Rutabaga
- Wasabi
- Watercress

In addition to supporting the growth of beneficial bacteria in the gut, Brassica family vegetables have been shown to enhance cellular detoxification. The liver is not the only location where detoxification is ongoing. We now know that skin cells are equipped with an elaborate detoxification system called *phase 2*, and certain chemicals within Brassica vegetables have been shown to support this system. For example, broccoli sprouts are rich in a chemical called sulforaphane, and its topical application protects skin cells against UV damage. Oral consumption of broccoli sprouts maintains higher levels of the powerful skin-protecting antioxidant CoQ_{10} and decreases body-wide markers of oxidative stress.

Because Japan is home to the oldest living people on Earth, researchers have spent quite a bit of time studying the genetics, diet, and lifestyle of the Japanese. Undoubtedly, many aspects of the Japanese diet may promote longevity and healthy skin through the aging process. Since intestinal microflora have been theorized to influence the aging process, it would be interesting to note any major differences between the intestinal microflora of Japanese and North American adults. Researchers from the University of Tokyo and the Ludwig Institute of Cancer in Toronto compared the fecal microflora of Japanese Tokyoites consuming a typical Japanese diet to that of healthy Toronto residents consuming a typical Western diet. As you may have imagined already, the levels of *Lactobacilli* and *Bifidobacteria* were significantly higher among the Japanese.

Looking even a little bit more deeply, researchers found that the overall levels of *Bifidobacteria* were much higher among rural dwellers of the Japanese region known for great longevity than among Tokyo adults. The levels of *Bifidobacteria* in the rural region, where residents adhere more strictly to the traditional Japanese diet, were higher than those of a Tokyo resident twenty years younger. *Bifidobacteria* levels usually drop through the aging process, and some consider levels of this bacteria to be a reliable marker of aging.

Note that rural Japanese are the least likely to use conventional and microwave ovens. Foods, even meats and fish, are prepared with water on a regular basis so the preformed AGE content is almost certainly lower among these residents. The bottom line is that a more healthy profile of intestinal bacteria is associated with longevity, which is in turn associated with fewer processed foods, more fiber, and fewer AGE-containing foods.

Probiotics and UV Protection

In earlier chapters, we discussed at length how UV radiation from the sun (and other sources) is the scourge of the skin-aging process. Older Japanese and Russian research suggests that the external administration of probiotic bacteria can help prevent radiation-induced sickness. One of the reasons we can get sick very easily, and even develop cancer, after prolonged sun exposure is that radiation suppresses our immune system. After prolonged sun exposure, we are not in a good position to fight and our immune defense lines are certainly weakened.

In a study published in the *European Journal of Dermatology* (2008), Swiss researchers showed that an orally consumed strain of *Lactobacillus* can lead to a quick return of normal immune functioning in adult volunteers after UV exposure. The prevention of immune suppression and rapid restoration of skin and body-wide immune defense upon UV exposure had been demonstrated previously in animals supplemented with probiotics. A separate study in the same journal showed that *Lactobacillus casei* (Dannon's DanActive) could specifically reduce skin inflammation when added to animal food.

Researchers from the University of Texas did not find statistically significant differences in skin-cancer rates among animals fed various levels of dried yogurt powder, although they did note trends indicating protection because the animals consuming the highest percentage of yogurt powder in their diets maintained the lowest incidence of skin carcinomas. The carcinoma incidence was three times higher in the animals with no yogurt powder in the diet, so more research is due in this area.

Probiotics and Ceramides

As mentioned, fermented milk has enjoyed a rich history as a beautifying agent. Going back to ancient Egypt, fermented milk was used topically on the skin to promote beauty. We now know that sour milk provides an excellent source of lactic acid, a well-established natural exfoliant. Topical lactic acid and other so-called alpha-hydroxy acids (AHA) can undoubtedly improve the appearance of aged skin. Research shows that exfoliation via AHA can provide a smooth appearance, decrease areas of hyperpigmentation, and make wrinkles appear less deep to observers. However, there may be more to the ancient sour milk therapy than just the lactic acid.

Italian researchers have recently shown that topical yogurt bacteria can help manufacture the ceramides in human epidermis. Remember the ceramides? They are the lipids that make up the mortar of the "brick wall" in the stratum corneum. More ceramides equals more moisture retained in a well-hydrated skin. Indeed, a recent human study of the yogurt-derived bacterial products showed a significant improvement in ceramide levels of the stratum corneum and enhanced skin-hydration levels.

Korean researchers reported in 2005 that probiotics produce natural chemicals that, when topically applied, limit the growth of undesirable, inflammation-promoting skin bacteria. In addition, topically applied *Bifidobacteria*-fermented soy milk improved elasticity of the skin and increased the glycosaminoglycan (GAG) content of the dermis in animals and in adults after three months. The Japanese study, published in the *Journal of Cosmetic Science* (2004), clearly shows that we have much to learn about probiotics, fermented products, and their influence on human skin.

> In addition to yogurt and probiotic supplements, one way to boost beneficial bacteria may be a daily cup of java. A study in the *International Journal of Food Microbiology* (2009) showed that adult volunteers who consumed three cups of coffee daily for twenty-one days significantly improved gut levels of healthy *Bifidobacteria*.

Stress and Intestinal Bacteria

In chapter 1, we introduced the notion that stress may drive the early development of visible signs of aging. For example, a history of a pessimistic mental outlook and depressive symptoms can add four years onto the facial aging of older women as perceived by others. Most adults understand, and research certainly shows, that stress is a major contributor to modern illnesses. Chronic stress can compromise health for many reasons, and one of these reasons, the loss of beneficial intestinal microflora, just doesn't seem to get the respect it deserves. Research has shown that psychological and physical stressors have a considerable negative impact on beneficial intestinal bacteria. Indeed, one may consider stress to be a potent eliminator of our good *Lactobacilli* and *Bifidobacteria*.

When adults are sick, such as with colds and flu, intestinal *Lactobacillus* is depleted. The same is true of overindulgence in alcohol. Also, anger and fear can increase undesirable intestinal bacteria strains by almost tenfold. These are the same strains of bacteria that have recently been linked with obesity.

STRESSED COSMONAUTS

The first solid stress-microflora studies were conducted by Russian scientists who were closely monitoring a group of cosmonauts preparing for space flight. In the days leading up to the launch, as nervous-emotional stressors were reported to be higher, the researchers found a coincidental decrease in *Lactobacilli* and *Bifidobacteria* levels. The *Bifidobacteria* appeared to be extremely vulnerable to preflight emotional stress.

Even after the flight, the microflora remained altered, with increases in less desirable species and long-term depletion of beneficial bacteria. In addition to preflight emotional stress affecting the good bacteria, additional experimental studies showed that the flight conditions, including the stress of restraint and confinement, lead to significant decreases in *Lactobacilli* and *Bifidobacteria*.

Endurance athletes who exercise intensely to exhaustion have also been reported to have lower levels of *Bifidobacteria*. Athletes who work to near exhaustion frequently report gastrointestinal complaints, which may be due to stress-induced alterations in the intestinal microflora. Exam stress can also lower the levels of our good bacteria, as found in a study involving undergraduate students taking exams.

Numerous other reports from animal studies show that stress can alter the intestinal microflora. Overcrowding and excessive heat can increase less desirable bacteria and decrease *Lactobacilli*. Noise stress and a feeling of being trapped will lower *Lactobacilli* in laboratory animals. Psychological stress encourages the growth of yeasts in animals, an overgrowth that can be inhibited with the anti-anxiety medication Xanax (alprazolam). Remarkably, taking a drug known to limit anxiety and reactivity to stress appears to limit changes in the intestinal microflora.

The effects of intestinal bacteria may even extend to human behavior itself. This is important because a bad mood plus high stress equals wrinkles. Among primates, maternal stress during pregnancy can result in a reduction of both *Lactobacilli* and *Bifidobacterium* concentrations. In the offspring, measures of infant independence are correlated with infant *Lactobacilli* and *Bifidobacteria*. In other words, the infant primates with higher *Lactobacillus* and *Bifidobacteria* species were more independent and exploratory than those with low levels of friendly bacteria. Lower *Lactobacilli* levels have been specifically correlated with the display of stress-indicative behaviors in animals.

A new University of Toronto study published in the journal *Gut Pathogens* (2009) has shown that oral administration of the Yakult *Lactobacillus casei* strain Shirota can reduce clinical anxiety in adult patients with chronic fatigue syndrome. Stress-related reductions in *Lactobacilli* and psychological stress itself can make the intestine more permeable to undesirable material. This means higher inflammation and greater potential damage to your skin over time. While scientists figure out the precise mechanisms behind the stress-induced alterations to the intestinal microflora, it is clear that the consumption of probiotic bacteria may be advisable during times of stress.

SPLENDA AND YOUR GUT

New research by a team from Duke University shows that the artificial sweetener sucralose (better known by North Americans as *Splenda*) can change the intestinal acid-alkaline balance and significantly reduce the friendly bacteria such as *Bifidobacteria and Lactobacillus* in the gut. Consider a report in *Environmental Science & Technology* (2008) indicating that excreted sucralose persists in the environment, and water treatment plants can do little to remove it. In short, you may be consuming sucralose without even knowing it.

Look East, Far East

Let's review for a moment, because up to this point we have covered a fair amount of nutritional ground. We have described how a variety of deeply colored fruits and vegetables, whole grains, healthy fats, fish, seafood, and culinary herbs may protect against the visible signs of aging. We have made claim that too much sugar and fructose and too many foods prepared on high and dry heat can add to the skin's internal glycation, or AGE, load. We have argued that the gut and its resident bacteria, specifically *Lactobacillus* and *Bifidobacteria*, may play an underestimated role in the aging of human skin.

If there was a lick of truth to our contention that diet matters when it comes to the aging of human skin, then surely we would see differences in nations that have a relatively stellar diet. So if you still don't believe that a healthy diet has a substantial connection to skin health, let's look at an exemplary cultural example, the Japanese. We mentioned earlier in this chapter that the Japanese are the oldest lived people on Earth, and although Japanese nutrition is sadly changing for the worse, the Japanese still maintain a diet for Westerners to envy. Because of this, Japanese skin, at least to some degree, is protected against the visible signs of aging by nutritional insulation.

An observational study showed that North American females aged twenty-nine to sixty-nine were much more likely to experience an earlier onset of facial wrinkles and sagging than women of the same age from Tokyo. Even within Asian nations, differences exist in the visible signs of aging. A recent study in the *Journal of Dermatological Science* (2007) shows internation differences in the severity of wrinkles through the aging process. Among close to one hundred women residing in each of three Asian cities (Tokyo, Japan; Shanghai, China; Bangkok, Thailand), the residents of Tokyo had the least visible signs of skin aging. In particular, there were major differences in the visible signs of aging between Tokyo and Bangkok residents. Women living in Bangkok were more likely to show early wrinkles and sagging. Once again, the researchers did not bother to gather data on history of smoking or sun exposure. However, since Bangkok lies closer to the equator, UV exposure is likely to play a role.

Now that we know the aging of the participants' skin actually is different, we can analyze differences in regional diets. Surprisingly, diet wasn't even mentioned as a potential factor in either of the two comparison studies (North America vs. Japan and inter-Asian studies). But with our nutritional vision, we see massive differences in the North American diet versus that of Japan. We can also make a strong argument for diet as a factor between Tokyo and Bangkok.

Looking first at the differences between the North American diet and that of the Japanese, the graphs that follow show that the one hundred or so adults found to have an earlier onset of the visible signs of facial aging would be much more likely to consume a diet with massive quantities of sugar, vegetable oils (especially soybean oil; we love the oil and avoid the soybeans themselves while the Japanese avoid the oil and eat the skin-protective soybeans), meat, and milk. In contrast, the Japanese women would have been much more likely to have consumed a long-term diet high in fish and seafood, vegetables, and legumes.

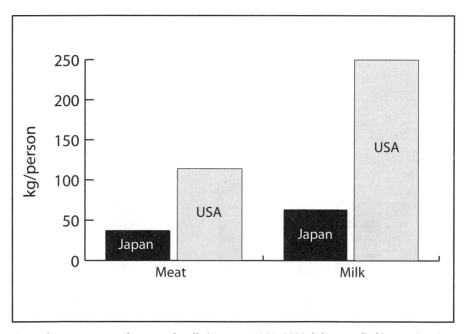

Annual consumption of meat and milk (average, 1980–2000; kilograms [kg]/person/year).

Some glaring differences in the diets between Japan and Thailand also pertain to skin aging. As the graphs show, the Tokyoites, with fewer wrinkles and less sagging, would likely consume three times more fish and seafood, almost three times more vegetables, and far more soybeans than the Thai

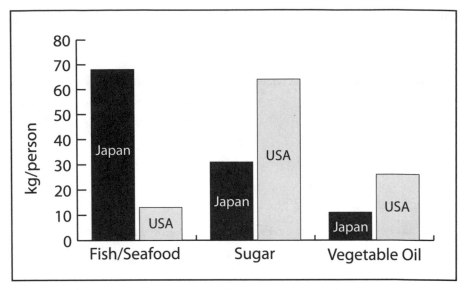

Annual consumption of fish/seafood, sugar, and vegetable oil (average, 1980–2000; kg/person/year).

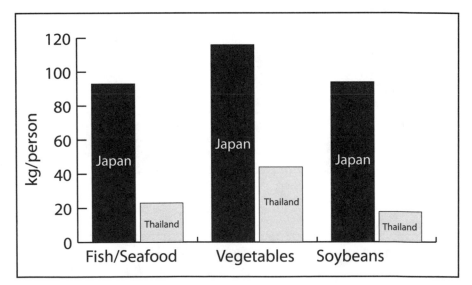

Annual consumption of fish/seafood, vegetables, and soybeans (average, 1980–2000; kg/person/year).

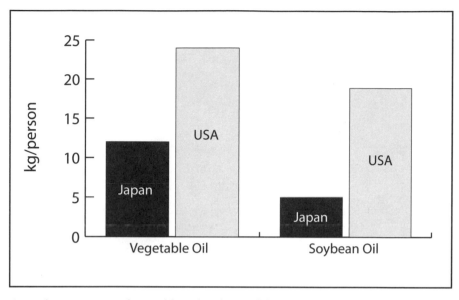

Annual consumption of vegetable and soybean oil (average, 1980–2000; kg/person/year).

participants. Differences in healthy food consumption between Japan and China are marginal, as were the differences in visible signs of aging. The only real edge belongs to the Japanese, who consume about three times more fish and seafood than the Chinese.

To be very clear, we are not stating that diet is the only—or even the largest—factor in the early development of visible signs of aging among North American females, as compared to their Japanese counterparts. To be fair, middle-aged or older Japanese women can often be seen walking or riding bikes while using umbrellas and facial visors to block out UV rays. This practice is very rare among the young, and combined with major changes to dietary practices in Japan in recent years, as well as the massive use of wireless technology, only time will tell if the early onset of visible signs of aging will become more apparent.

Some researchers like to write findings off to genetics. That old song and dance was tried in 1964 when large-scale research showed that the rates of acne in Japan were half those of North American teens. The genetic card sounded good at the time; however, the rates of acne in Japan and the

United States have recently become indistinguishable, yet genetics have not changed. Acne rates have increased as the young Japanese have moved away from traditional eating habits and begun reporting higher levels of stress. Therefore, the aging manifestations may be evident in the not-too-distant future.

5

The Brain-Skin Connection
and Your Beauty Sleep

"The skin is often hit hard by nervous strain, anxiety, worry, shock, overload. To meet such tension factors and thus influence the root of the skin trouble, the following general (stress-management) suggestions are as important as any medical prescription."

THIS IS FROM THE SAME FUNDAMENTALS *of Medical Dermatology* textbook (1942) that we quoted earlier. As we are sure you will agree, the textbook authors' recommendations and techniques to reduce stress (or as they called it, tension) for healthier skin are every bit as applicable to our lives as they were all those years ago. Indeed, the recommendations are the very foundation of the modern-day mind-body medicine modalities that we will consider.

Until recently, dermatology as a profession has been lax in underscoring the importance of stress, tension, and lifestyle factors in skin conditions. Much like nutrition, such influences seemed non-scientific and fell out of favor for many years. Thankfully, the refocusing on stress, sleep, and a healthy lifestyle for the maintenance of glowing skin is now accompanied by elegant research studies, investigations that prove a very intimate connection between our brain and emotions and our skin structure and functioning. Before we ponder the specific details and benefits of stress reduction and sleep hygiene, it is important to examine how and why stress is so destructive to radiant, glowing skin.

What Is Stress?

Over the years, a collection of human and animal studies, as well as physician reports, have linked psychological stress to virtually every skin condition. From atopic dermatitis to psoriasis, from acne to skin cancer, stress is a trigger or exacerbating factor.

Stress can be defined as the thoughts, feelings, behaviors, and physiological changes that occur when the demands placed upon a person exceed his or her perceived ability to cope. Stress-related thoughts, feelings, behaviors, and physical bodily changes are ultimately influenced by demands and perceptions.

Since we don't want to break with tradition, let's get the obligatory "Not all stress is bad" statement out of the way. Yes, some amount of stress can improve performance and even inoculate us against future stress and improve resiliency. Clearly, we can't live in a stress-free bubble, and adversities in life can certainly make us stronger. However, since the average North American reportedly experiences about fifty brief stress response episodes per day— daily hassles, as they are called—we are not living in an age where lack of stress is a major health concern. It is also important to point out that stress need not always be related to overwork and too many social responsibilities. Boredom, lack of purpose, and loneliness can be extremely stressful.

The Skin Aging–Stress Connection

At the heart of the skin aging–stress connection lies the stress hormone called cortisol. Chronic elevation of this hormone is like acid rain to your collagen. The hormone has short-term health advantages (for example, immune support) during a legitimate crisis. However, when elevated on a chronic basis in the face of stress and anxiety-provoking environments, cortisol is associated with inflammation, increased oxidative stress, and other skin-assaulting forces.

Cortisol levels are 34 percent higher in those with chronic anxiety, and 36 percent higher in those with chronically elevated blood pressure as compared to healthy, non-stressed controls. Teachers who report high work stress have more than 20 percent higher cortisol on a regular basis, and associations have been noted between anger and higher cortisol among employees. In general, workers who report excessive commitments, time constraints in the face of daily assignments, and postponement of recreation due to workload have significantly higher cortisol levels.

DAILY HASSLES AND YOUR SKIN

In a landmark study published in the journal *Psychophysiology* (2007), those adults who reported a better mood, less stress, and more events perceived as uplifting had significantly lower levels of inflammatory chemicals. In contrast, those otherwise healthy adults who perceived a life filled with more stress, in the form of daily hassles over the previous month, had significantly higher blood levels of inflammatory chemicals.

A joint team from Kings College, London, and the University of Kansas recently showed much slower healing of the skin in adults who perceived the highest levels of stress. These were healthy adults, yet once again, a greater reporting of day-to-day worries was associated with higher cortisol, and the cortisol increase was clearly linked to poor healing of biopsy wounds through the skin. Other investigative groups have found that adults who have difficulty with anger control have higher levels of cortisol and longer wound-healing time. These studies are relevant to aging skin because one of the important features of proper wound healing is the reshaping and restructuring of normal collagen patterns.

Cortisol is released as part of the stress "response," a term for the automatic physiological changes and accompanying thoughts that occur in the event of a threat to our perceived safety. This doesn't have to be a matter of an actual threat to safety; note the word "perceived," and "safety" in this case is very broadly defined. A perceived threat to safety encompasses anything from being stuck in traffic to potential embarrassment in a work setting. Where we run into trouble is in the *perception* part of the equation. Our perception of danger, and ultimately the degree and style of reactivity to the "threats," are intricately related to our real and perceived coping abilities. Once demands start piling up beyond a level where we feel we can cope, when our true coping abilities are built like a shaky house of cards, and when acute becomes chronic, the path of dermal destruction is switched into high gear.

The damaging influence of stress is one additional mediator that can influence our genetic expression. Recall our discussion in chapter 1 that while we have a set of genetic cards at birth, our diet, toxic exposures, lifestyle, beliefs, stressors, and subsequent mental outlook can all influence genetic expression—meaning that the degree to which we experience an illness, or whether we experience an illness at all, may be dictated in part by external or so-called environmental factors. This is beautifully illustrated by the work of Elissa Epel, PhD, and colleagues from the University of California, San Francisco, who showed that both the perception and the chronic nature of stress can cause cells to age prematurely and die. In this groundbreaking 2004 study, women with the highest levels of perceived stress had markers of cellular longevity that indicated accelerated aging—and not just a little, the markers were equivalent to a *decade* or more of additional aging, compared to the low-stress group.

Stress later in life is not the only stress that causes the aging process to be more visible in the form of illness. Neal Krause, PhD, of the University of Michigan Institute of Gerontology, showed that a more frequent experience of traumatic life events in the younger years of life is highly predictive of ill health among seniors. The acid rain of cortisol is falling hard even at twenty and thirty years old, so don't think for a moment that the stressors of a difficult workplace and such are not eroding your dermal structure.

Mechanisms of Destruction

We have spent a decent portion of our discussion in previous chapters underscoring the reality that oxidative stress and inflammation are primary drivers of the skin-aging process. Psychological stress cannot be quarantined from any true discussion of inflammation, oxidative stress, and indeed, even gastrointestinal function and glycation. Chronic stress fires up a cascade of physiological events that promote the inflammatory chemicals that then promote collagen destruction.

Stress influences nearly every aspect of skin aging we have discussed thus far. For example, the collagen-destroying inflammatory chemical called PGE2 from chapter 2 is known to be elevated with chronic stress. MMPs responsible for breaking down collagen also may become overactive with stress. (Research shows elevated levels of MMPs in cancer patients with the highest depressive outlook.) Chronic stress, anxiety, and depressive symptoms are all associated with the increased generation of free radicals. This only serves to add to an already massive burden on the skin's antioxidant reserves.

Furthermore, the bacterial microflora of the intestines undergo significant change with chronic stress and anxiety. Intestinal permeability and an overgrowth of bacteria in the small intestine set the stage for an additional burden of unwanted material gaining access to the body-wide circulation. As reported recently in the *International Journal of Clinical Practice* (2008), patients with higher symptoms of chronic anxious and depressive thoughts are much more likely to have small intestinal bacterial overgrowth. This only serves to interfere with the absorption of much-needed antioxidants and anti-inflammatory nutrients.

Chronic stress and its accompanying cortisol elevations are also strongly associated with cardiovascular disease and the blockage of blood vessels. This is not without consequence to the skin because the stress-induced reduction of blood flow compromises the delivery of much-needed nutrients to, and the removal of toxic byproducts from, the skin layers.

We have referred to cortisol as acid rain in the dermis because it specifically inhibits both collagen and the glycosaminoglycan (GAG) production. When synthetic cortisol-like chemicals hit the market in 1949, they were the wonder drug of the century, right up there with antibiotics. There is no disputing that the advent of synthetic glucocorticoids changed medicine and improved the quality of life for millions. The glucocorticoids have great anti-inflammatory properties, and the drugs quickly became part of the arsenal against asthma, arthritis, and inflammatory skin conditions.

As with most drugs, getting a true handle on the side effects took time. Eventually, however, researchers figured out that topical glucocorticoids took a toll on the skin when they were used for long periods. The toll, in the case of long-term glucocorticoid use, was skin atrophy. The dermis becomes thinned out and rete ridges, which normally increase the blood flow to the epidermis, are lost. In essence the process is somewhat reflective of the skin-aging process. By the early 1960s, it had become quite evident that the glucocorticoids were inhibiting the production of collagen. Later, researchers determined that the scaffolding to the scaffolding, the GAGs, were also suffering at the hands of the glucocorticoid.

More recently, researchers discovered that the glucocorticoids actually influence collagen production negatively at the genetic level by sending out signals to the specific genes involved in collagen synthesis and breakdown. You might think that if signals to slow down collagen production are being sent by stress hormones like cortisol, then surely the MMPs that break down collagen would at least slow down—but they don't. The MMPs are busy breaking down collagen while its production has ground to a halt.

We are not addressing the issue of synthetic glucocorticoid use here; an individual who might need the prescription drugs has plenty of pros and cons to consider. The point of the discussion is to demonstrate the almost certain result of constantly bathing your skin cells in stress hormones—skin atrophy, collagen loss, fragility, and dermal wasting. Also, as a matter of clarity, cortisol does have acute anti-inflammatory properties. However, over time and with chronic stress, we become less responsive to them and the pendulum swings the other way, leaving unbridled inflammation.

The stress-induced assault to normal skin structure and function is not confined to the dermis. Psychological stress can compromise the barrier function of the skin. In other words, stress compromises the integrity of the stratum corneum in the epidermis, and this translates into a greater risk of dry, dehydrated skin. In one study, the skin barrier was more significantly impaired in students during stressful exam periods. And in a separate study, the stress of interviews disrupted skin-barrier function.

More recently, a study in *Psychosomatic Medicine* (2007) showed that speech preparation and delivery, as well as stress-provoking, complex mathematical tasks can impair skin-barrier function. Dermatological researchers from Cornell University have shown that stress-induced changes in the skin-barrier function are highly associated with blood levels of inflammatory chemicals: more stress equals more inflammatory chemicals, which equal compromised barrier function and water loss from the skin. Experimental studies show that stress interferes with the production of the fatty components of the stratum corneum.

> In simple terms, stress halts the manufacture of the mortar in your brick-and-mortar structure. The end result is a malformed brick wall that allows greater permeability of the wall and much greater water loss.

The same chain of events occurs when epidermal cells are bathed in synthetic stress hormones. Glucocorticoids also shut down the production of mortar for the stratum corneum. But, topical application of certain fats and ceramides can minimize the loss of barrier function in the presence of glucocorticoids. Also, topical application of citrus antioxidants (bioflavonoids) can negate most of the detrimental, collagen-destroying effect of glucocorticoids when both are applied together.

So all is not lost, and as we will discuss in some detail, nutrition and stress are a two-way street. Stress cannot be addressed in isolation from nutrition, any more than nutrition can be viewed in isolation from the lifestyle and day-to-day experiences of an individual. Stress changes dietary habits, and dietary habits themselves may contribute to stress in a protective or detrimental way.

Stressed Out

At this point, there should be no doubt that stress has short- and long-term consequences to the appearance of skin. Over the short term, epidermal skin-barrier function is altered, increasing the risk of dry, rough, and scaly skin. Over the long haul, loss of collagen and GAGs and structural changes can contribute to the visible signs of aging.

If you still don't believe the skin aging–stress connection, simply look at the before-inauguration and after-term pictures of previous presidents of the United States, and the connection will be self-evident. Some estimate that every year in office ages a president's body at a rate twice that of the normal per-year average.

As North Americans, we believe ourselves to be more stressed out than ever before, which makes that our reality. In recent years, the American Psychological Association has conducted an annual *Stress in America* survey, and it certainly indicates a rise in stress over the past five years. Half of all Americans report that stress has a negative impact on their personal and professional quality of life. Of those who are stressed, about half have sleep problems or consume unhealthy foods and extra calories as a means to combat stress or do both. Prescription-drug use for anxiety and depression is at an all-time high, with one in ten women taking antidepressants linked to facial wrinkling. Incredibly, one of every three doctor's visits by women in 2002 involved the patient walking out the door with a prescription for an antidepressant.

The increasing complexity of modern life, a move away from rural dwellings, and techno-stress are likely major driving forces of our increased perception of stress. Research has shown that rates of mental-health disorders are higher among city dwellers (and, by the way, oxidative stress burdens are higher due to pollution), and the blurring of the lines between work and family time have been shown to add stress. Time was when coworkers would only call others at home if it was a matter of the very survival of the company—not so today with crackberries, email, and cell phones. The technological advances mean that workin' for the man never stops. Research from the University of Glasgow indicates that the sheer bulk of emails employees must deal with are not only a major distraction, but also a significant source of stress.

Additional research in the *Journal of Marriage and Family* (2005) shows that cell phone use is linked to heightened psychological distress and reduced family satisfaction. Work spills over into the home, and ultimately the quality of life of the worker and those around him or her will suffer. According to a study in the *Journal of Occupational Health Psychology* (2005), employees who take their work home feel more exhausted and irritable when they finally have downtime at home.

IS YOUR CELL PHONE WRINKLING YOUR SKIN?

Scientists Paolo Giacomoni, PhD, and Glen Rein, PhD, were the first to report that electromagnetic frequency (EMF) exposure should be considered as a factor in the aging of human skin. Writing in the journal *Biogerontology* (2001), the researchers suggested that the massive increase in exposure to EMF in recent years, particularly through wireless devices and cell phones, may be driving the inflammatory processes in human skin. Case reports started showing up in the medical literature connecting landline base cordless phone use and skin cancer.

In 2003, researchers showed that when cell phone EMF exposure was applied along with UV radiation in animals there was an increased speed in the cancer process once skin cancer was initiated. Following this, researchers from Turkey published two separate studies, one in the *Journal of Dermatology* (2004) and the other in *Toxicology and Industrial Health* (2004), with both showing that exposure to cell-phone radiation in animals for 30 minutes per day caused significant oxidative stress in the skin. In addition, after ten days of 30-minute exposure, there was a significant thinning of the epidermis, alterations to the stratum corneum, and alteration to the collagen structures. The good news is that when antioxidants were added to the laboratory chow, the influence of the cell-phone EMF was minimized.

More recently, in the journal *BMC Genomics* (2008), researchers from Finland showed that cell phone EMF exposure for one hour caused changes in proteins within the skin of otherwise healthy human volunteers. This was the first indication that cell phone EMF exposure might influence skin health at the genetic level. When combined with the increase in facial melanoma among young adults, that finding suggests that wireless communication might be combining with UV exposure to damage our skin. Now, perhaps more than ever before, we need dietary protection for our skin.

Then, we have the cell phone–insomnia connection. At least three human studies have shown that cell-phone use close to bedtime can compromise the quality and depth of sleep. One of the more recent studies connected cell-phone use to insomnia, headaches, and mood-related symptoms the next day when used the night before. Specifically, the cell phone radiation interferes with the portion of sleep known to assist in rejuvenating and repairing the

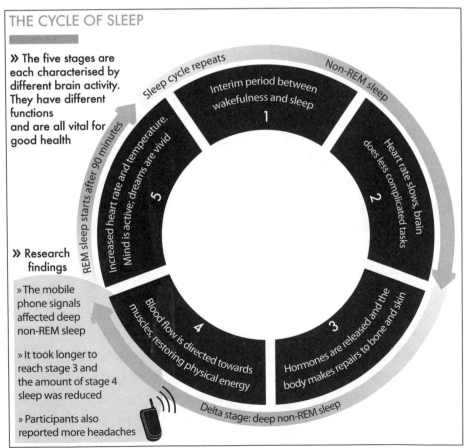

THE CYCLE OF SLEEP

» The five stages are each characterised by different brain activity. They have different functions and are all vital for good health

» Research findings

» The mobile phone signals affected deep non-REM sleep

» It took longer to reach stage 3 and the amount of stage 4 sleep was reduced

» Participants also reported more headaches

Sleep cycle repeats

Non-REM sleep

Interim period between wakefulness and sleep
1

Heart rate slows, brain does less complicated tasks
2

Hormones are released and the body makes repairs to bone and skin
3

Delta stage: deep non-REM sleep

Blood flow is directed towards muscles, restoring physical energy
4

Increased heart rate and temperature. Mind is active; dreams are vivid
5

REM sleep starts after 90 minutes

GRAPHIC: Charlotte Braunagel

SOURCES: The EM Academy | IoS research

mind and body from the daily grind. Wireless use may also be lowering the sleep hormone melatonin. In our context, we have concerns that more and more adults are not getting their beauty sleep. Considering that the use of prescription sleeping pills has increased threefold over the last decade among those aged eighteen to twenty-four, a group that ordinarily sleeps well, something obviously is driving the sleep issues. Genetics haven't changed.

Why Beauty Sleep?

The importance of sleep for a youthful, glowing, and vibrant appearance is beyond obvious. Extended TV and video game use, and sleep deprivation in general, makes us look tired, particularly around the eyes. Everyone knows that occasional sleep deprivation makes us look haggard and rough for a day or so. It seems harmless enough when it is short-lived. Yet when inadequate sleep becomes society's norm, we have a major problem with the promotion of the skin-aging process.

Sleep is a time for skin repair and rejuvenation. Sleep deprivation impairs the normal process of healing in skin wounds. Since chronic stress can impair sleep, and sleep deprivation can also promote stress, it shouldn't be surprising that a number of studies have shown sleep deprivation to also be associated with inflammation and oxidative stress. A study in the *Journal of Investigative Dermatology* (2001) showed that women who are deprived of sleep have disturbed skin-barrier function, greater water loss from the skin, and a far higher level of inflammatory chemicals in circulation.

Over time, the chronic loss of beauty sleep will do more than just disturb the outer epidermal layers. The inflammatory chemicals will eventually take a toll on the deeper dermal structures. Deep beauty sleep is a time when collagen-damaging cortisol is normally kept in check, yet those with consistent sleep loss are known to have much higher levels of the stress hormone.

Much like the gut and the skin, the brain and the skin seem so far removed from each other that major physiological links between the two may be difficult to comprehend, including those pertaining to sleep. Yet, early in fetal development, the nervous system and skin share the same embryological cells called the embryonic ectoderm. We are now learning that "brain" neurotransmitters and hormones are not exclusive to the brain at all. The skin and central nervous system share similar hormones, neurotransmitters (chemical messengers), and respective receptors that work like a lock and key to bring about physiological changes. Recently, scientists have discovered that the skin is reliant upon two "brain" chemicals with anti-aging properties—melatonin and gamma-aminobutyric acid (GABA). Levels of both of these chemicals are lower in adults with chronic sleep loss.

Why is this a significant problem for the visible signs of aging? A lack of GABA in the skin is associated with diminished collagen and GAGs, and impaired barrier function. On the other hand, GABA application enhances the survival of the cells that make collagen and the important GAG hyaluronic acid, even when under oxidative stress. The 30 percent lower GABA levels experienced by those with chronic insomnia are almost certainly not without consequence to the skin.

Melatonin has antioxidant and anti-inflammatory properties in the skin. A long-term lack of melatonin may have a detrimental influence on collagen structure in the dermis and may cause thinning of epidermal barrier structures. Melatonin and GABA almost certainly are important players in the repair and rejuvenation processes of beauty sleep.

There is yet one more reason to get your beauty sleep—maintaining healthy gut microflora. We have been harping on the gut-skin connection and have discussed in some detail the knowledge that stress alters gut bacteria. Sleep deprivation can cause a more permeable intestinal lining, which in turn allows unwanted material access to the bloodstream.

In 2008, researchers from Japan's National Institute of Mental Health reported that greater waking through the night and overall loss of sleep time is associated with the loss of—yes, our *Bifidobacteria*. Those who were observed to have both sleep abnormalities and reported irregular bowel function had only half the *Bifidobacteria* levels of the healthy control subjects.

Sleep deprivation is known to be associated with subsequent gastrointestinal complaints, and as outlined in chapter 4, any loss of healthy bacteria for whatever reason is not good. Inflammation, oxidative stress, and glycation may ensue.

SLEEP HABITS

- Bedroom should be as dark as possible for maximum melatonin release.
- Bedroom should be used for sleeping only. Remove the television and the computer.
- Bedroom environment should be organized and free of clutter to be an oasis from the rest of the world.
- Bedroom temperature should be comfortable. Too much heat or cold interferes with sleep.
- Keep a regular schedule; go to bed at the same time, even on weekends.
- Eliminate caffeine-containing beverages and food after 4 p.m.
- Perform exercise in the daytime or early evening.
- Alcohol should not be used as a sleep aid.
- Avoid eating large meals late at night.
- For nourishment before bed, go with warm milk and a small piece of whole-grain toast.
- Use relaxation techniques, such as meditation, in the evening.
- Invest in a comfortable mattress.
- Earplugs and soundproofing may help some, while others respond to a steady noise device, such as a waterfall or ocean sounds.
- Avoid TV news and action movies before bed. They can increase stress hormones, anxiety, and worry.

Sleepless in America

North Americans are definitely in debt with a sleep deficit that has been building over the years. Stress-induced sleep problems are a big part of the picture, and wireless communication, computers, evening lights, and TVs can reduce our sleep-inducing melatonin levels. Today, more than one-third of Americans sleep fewer than 6.5 hours per night, yet just a century ago, the average night's sleep was nine hours. Children of all ages are sleeping one to two hours less than what they require each night.

A 2008 study by the U.S. Center for Disease Control and Prevention reports that 70 percent of adults perceive that they are not getting adequate sleep on a daily basis. Overall, we have shaved off an average of 1.5 hours of sleep per night in relation to one hundred years ago.

Don't be fooled by the notion that only four or five hours of sleep are required. While proponents of such nonsense usually cite a famous historical figure who hardly slept, research shows otherwise. Adults who sleep five or fewer hours per night have a 15 percent higher chance of dying early from any cause—cardiovascular, cancer, you name it. The bottom line is that a consistent lack of sleep ages the body, and it ages the skin. Just like stress itself, sleep deprivation causes us to change our dietary habits.

Not Reaching for Kale and Broccoli

Stress and sleep deprivation undoubtedly change all good intentions about healthy eating. While some respond to stress by skipping meals, most of us gravitate toward overeating or consuming foods and beverages that are no friend to the skin, or doing both. Certainly, we don't reach for the spinach when stress and sleep deprivation are the norm. Popeye is the only exception to that rule.

> Both acute and chronic stressors have the potential to negatively influence our food choices, which, in turn, can promote the cycle of skin aging.

Even those who under-eat during stress report an increase in snacking on foods rich in sugar and unhealthy fats. Like fool's gold, fats and sugars provide a very brief palatable comfort. However, when used to combat stress and fatigue, they spike insulin and produce glycation and inflammation of the skin.

VEGETABLE DIP

A variety of studies have shown that stress influences dietary choices. Corporate workers approaching deadlines, students during exam periods, and nurses and teachers under stress have all been shown to change their dietary habits. The common thread is greater fast-food consumption and higher intakes of sweets, total fat, and overall calories and fat. Intake of fruits and vegetables takes a very noticeable dip during times of stress.

Sleep restriction also influences how we eat. Karine Spiegel, PhD, and colleagues from the University of Chicago showed that not only does sleep restriction increase hunger, it also drives us to consume more sweets, starchy foods, and other high-carbohydrate, high-calorie foods. Consumption of such foods increased by 33 to 45 percent in sleep-deprived individuals. In contrast, sleep deprivation did not push participants toward fruits, vegetables, or high-protein nutrients.

Other investigators have reported that those with sleep problems are more likely to eat at fast-food outlets and shun healthier fare cooked at home. The most recent Harvard study, in the *Journal of Clinical Sleep Medicine* (2008), showed that adults with sleep-disordered breathing are significantly more likely to consume excess total and saturated fat.

Tryptophan, Sleep, and Stress

The amino-acid tryptophan has a reputation for sedation, and it has long been known that tryptophan can be converted into the so-called feel-good brain chemical called serotonin. This conversion of tryptophan into serotonin requires certain vitamins, especially vitamin B$_6$, and is optimized in the presence of some carbohydrates. That's why so many people feel relaxed and sleepy when they finish the Thanksgiving meal. The tryptophan from the turkey gains access to the brain in the presence of sweet potatoes, stuffing, and cranberry sauce.

When scientists give adult volunteers test meals without tryptophan (the so-called tryptophan-depletion test), insomnia and poor depth of sleep has been shown to be a primary result. Indeed, the tryptophan-depletion test may also provoke anxiety and depressive symptoms. There is, however, yet one angle to the tryptophan story outside of the Thanksgiving turkey connection—stress-induced inflammation, or any sort of inflammation, interferes with the conversion of tryptophan into serotonin.

Over-activity of the stress branch of the nervous system—or the sympathetic branch, as it is known—is associated with over-eating, changes in blood hormones, and a decrease in blood levels of tryptophan. The rules of the tryptophan-conversion game are dramatically altered when inflammation is ongoing. When inflammatory chemicals are present, whether through skin inflammation or general stress-induced inflammation, the tryptophan is converted into a wasteful product called kynurenic acid. Don't worry about the biochemistry; the bottom line is that this is not good—and especially not good for the health of your collagen. Research shows that when tryptophan is depleted by inflammatory chemicals, the MMPs that break down your collagen go hog wild. Administration of tryptophan can help slow down the MMP activity, even in the presence of inflammatory chemicals.

> Tryptophan plays an important role in the skin, and depletion through stress, inflammation, and sleep deprivation will encourage the breakdown of collagen. In addition, tryptophan is converted into serotonin in the skin, and inadequate serotonin may compromise the skin barrier function in the epidermis.

Tryptophan also has a gut connection. You didn't think we could leave the intestinal microflora out of this story, did you? As discussed, chronic stress and impaired digestion can have a very detrimental influence on our beneficial intestinal bacteria and, by extension, on our inflammation-oxidative stress load. The plot thickens just a wee bit more, thanks to intriguing new research from Irish scientists. Investigators reported in the *Journal of Psychiatric Research* (2008) that animals consuming food with probiotics (*Bifidobacteria*) mixed within the chow (versus chow alone) had significantly higher blood levels of tryptophan and less breakdown of serotonin in the brain!

We also can't leave the tryptophan story without a mention of our omega-3-rich favorite, fish. Fish consumption can boost blood tryptophan levels much more than comparative meals of chicken or beef. Not only are the blood tryptophan levels higher after fish (versus similar portions of chicken or beef), but you also will most likely experience a greater sense of satiety (fullness) after fish consumption. More blood tryptophan translates into higher brain serotonin levels, elevated mood, and a feeling of satiety.

Foods and Nutrients for Stress

The relationship between nutrition and mental health has been grossly underappreciated. Omega-3 and other nutrient insufficiences are associated with altered mood states, anger, and depression. For example, some half-dozen studies have shown that both intra-nation and international fish and seafood consumption appears to be protective against depression, seasonal affective disorder (so-called winter blues), bipolar (manic) depression, and postpartum depression. The same anti-inflammatory eicosapentaenoic acid (EPA) omega-3 that is protecting your skin is also responsible for normal communication within and between nerve cells.

The direct nutritional influences on our resilience to stress and overall mental outlook are important as a means to prevent stress-induced damage to the skin. Omega-3 fatty acids can improve depressive symptoms in adults with depressive disorders. However, the mental-health benefits of taking dietary and supplemental omega-3 fatty acids may also extend to otherwise healthy adults. A study in the *European Journal of Clinical Investigation* (2005) showed that one month of fish oil (versus olive oil) supplementation improved both mood and mental functioning in otherwise healthy adults without an anxiety or depressive disorder.

Researchers also have shown that taking EPA-rich fish-oil capsules (versus a vegetable-oil placebo) daily for three months can decrease anger and anxiety levels. Researchers from the University of Pittsburgh showed that among 106 healthy adults, those with the lowest blood levels of omega-3 were most likely to report mild depressive symptoms and a more negative outlook on life, and to be more impulsive.

In the most recent study published in the *American Journal of Clinical Nutrition* (2009), Canadian researchers showed that EPA-rich fish oil lowered perceptions of psychological distress and depressive symptoms in women who did not actually meet depression criteria. Consider also that at least two human studies have shown that fish oil can lower cortisol levels when adults are subjected to laboratory stressors. The bottom line is that fish and seafood, as well as fish-oil supplements, may lift mood and help mitigate day-to-day perceptions of stress.

Whole-grain, fiber-rich cereals that are low in sugar are a friend to the skin. We covered this in some detail in chapter 1. Fiber reduces the likelihood of blood sugar and insulin spikes, as well as glycation in the skin. Fiber-rich cereals are nutrient-dense cereals, and many of the nutrients, particularly B vitamins stripped away from processed grains, can protect skin and mental outlook.

Andrew Smith, PhD, and colleagues from Cardiff University have shown that high-fiber (15 percent or more) breakfast cereal can reduce fatigue in adults, as compared to low-fiber cereals. Smith's study, published in the journal *Appetite* (2001), showed that high-fiber breakfast is associated with less fatigue and emotional distress, and fewer cognitive difficulties. More recently, Smith reported in a separate study that regular consumption of fibrous breakfast cereal is associated with lower levels of the stress hormone cortisol. Think about the 1930 Post Bran Flakes advertisement; turns out that a high-fiber, low-sugar cereal can improve energy, help keep stress in check, and turn off the acid-rain showers on your collagen after all.

Various nutrients have also been found to be important in maintaining a healthy mental outlook. Low blood levels of zinc, selenium, and folic acid have all been shown (individually) to be related to low mood states. Interestingly, each of these nutrients helps metabolize omega-3 fatty acids and boost omega-3 levels. Patients with mood disorders are known to have blood folate levels about 25 percent lower than adults without depression. Incredibly, low blood levels of folate before psychological interventions have been associated with a poor outcome with subsequent antidepressant therapies. Just 500 micrograms of supplemental folic acid improves depression and limits side effects when used with antidepressant medications.

Some of the other B vitamins—including vitamin B_3 (niacin and its derivatives), vitamin B_6, and vitamin B_2—are associated with behavioral and mood changes when dietary intake is sub-par. Vitamin B_3 helps in various mental health disorders, and administration of different forms of B_3 orally, topically, or both, has a long history of use in dermatology.

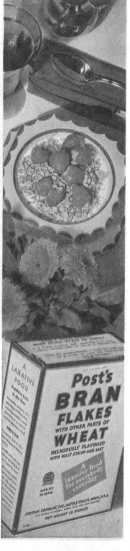

Your dining table can do damage your *dressing* table can't repair!

"THOSE tired-looking lines about my eyes —surely a touch of 'Eye Shadow' will hide them!

"That rather 'washed-out' look that has worried me of late —a whisper of rouge on the cheeks will make it right!"

Few women deceive themselves with such musings *nowadays!* They know that lasting beauty is more than skin-deep —*they pay as much attention to their dining tables as they do to their dressing tables!*

Nature is generous but jealous. She gives you the rose-petal loveliness of youth to keep just so long as you obey her—and no longer!

Break Nature's laws and how soon the penalty is apparent in your face! No wonder modern women take care

to protect themselves against that great beauty destroyer — *constipation.*

The Pleasant Daily Help toward Natural Beauty

Bran bulk in the daily diet aids Nature to rid the body of poisonous wastes that undermine beauty. And what more delicious way to take the daily portion of bran than in Post's Bran Flakes — which has made millions *like* bran.

With milk or cream, fruits or berries, in full-flavored, fluffy muffins—delicious! And, what is more important, *effective.* Tomorrow is an excellent time to begin Post's Bran Flakes.

Cases of recurrent constipation, due to insufficient bulk in the diet, should yield to Post's Bran Flakes. If your case is abnormal, consult a competent physician at once and follow his advice.

POST'S BRAN FLAKES

★ WITH OTHER PARTS OF WHEAT

© 1930, G. F. Corp.

A Product of General Foods Corporation

July 1930 Good Housekeeping

Post's Cereal Company informs consumers in *Good Housekeeping* magazine (1930) that unhealthy foods can take a toll on the skin, while fiber-rich foods help promote beauty from the inside-out. Modern research is validating the message.

Most recently, a study in the *Journal of Dermatology* (2008) shows that topical B_3 as niacinamide can reduce visible signs of aging, eye wrinkles in particular, in adult women. Vitamin B_6 is important for normal collagen production and skin-barrier function. Finally, vitamin B_2 (riboflavin) is essential for collagen production, and it, too, has been linked to human mood disorders when the body has an inadequate supply.

Zinc is a nutrient tied to the visible signs of aging. Blood zinc levels are lower in individuals with major depression. The connection between low levels of zinc in depression and low levels of zinc in acne are almost certainly not coincidental. Remember that of all vitamins and minerals, a diet consistently deficient in zinc is most closely linked to wrinkles and facial aging. Research shows just 25 milligrams of zinc daily can lead to significant improvement in depressive symptoms and enhance the effectiveness of antidepressant medications.

At least five studies have shown that low selenium levels are associated with a poor mood state, so it is important to recall that selenium is one of the most important allies in defense of aging skin. It is a critical nutrient in protection from UV radiation. Selenium supplementation can curb anxiety in those with a reported high psychological burden. In addition, a daily multivitamin can improve cognition and mood.

Chromium is yet another nutrient tied to both mental outlook and healthy skin. Best known for its ability to regulate blood-sugar levels and improve acne, it also acts as an antidepressant. Chromium supplementation can help alleviate depressive symptoms and carbohydrate cravings in depressed adults.

If you need an afternoon pick-me-up, think of green tea, arguably nature's most skin-friendly anti-stress beverage. The epigallocatechin gallate (EGCG) within green tea can help protect collagen, and it has underappreciated value for the stress system. This antioxidant polyphenol has been shown to lower the stress response by its actions on the GABA system in the brain. As mentioned, GABA is the major inhibitory brain chemical, acting like a set of brakes when we start to feel overwhelmed. It is called an inhibitory chemical because it helps us block out unneeded stimuli, damping down the system, and preventing overload.

Stress conditions deplete GABA levels. Recently, Japanese researchers found that 100 milligrams of naturally fermented GABA induce relaxation and reduce anxiety in a variety of stressful situations. Green tea is also particularly rich in an amino acid called L-theanine. Theanine stimulates GABA production as well as the feel-good neurotransmitter serotonin, which may be the reason for the lack of jitteriness after green tea, as opposed to an energy drink or coffee. You may be thinking that all this is well and good, but why does this make green tea a pick-me-up? Interestingly, a number of studies show that theanine promotes mental functioning yet also has anti-stress properties that calm the brain. Green tea seems to provide the perfect combination of GABA, theanine, and caffeine to provide the energy, mental focus, and sense of relaxation needed to deal with stressful days.

Mind-Body Medicine

The ill-conceived notion that mind and body are separate and distinct has lingered in medicine for centuries. Thankfully, this disconnect has been put to rest in recent years with an overwhelming amount of clinical research. Nowhere is the mind-body connection more painfully obvious than in the clinical response to placebos used in human studies. Skin conditions are not immune to a placebo response. Even in complex cases of acne and other inflammatory skin conditions, 30 or more percent of patients will get well on the look-a-like medicine that is merely a sugar pill or inert cream.

In a well-publicized 2008 review of many antidepressant drug trials, researchers concluded that there is little difference between antidepressant medications and placebos in clinical outcome. Obviously, individuals who *believe* they are taking a chemically active pill or herb can ultimately influence their own progression of illness or skin condition to a degree. Thanks to sophisticated brain-imaging studies, we know that the placebo response can actually change brain physiology. This placebo effect appears to be particularly strong in illnesses with a significant stress connection. The lesson from the placebo is simple yet profound: the mind has a significant effect on the course of illness.

In efforts to manage stress and combat the skin-aging process, the goal is to grab the thought processes and lessons of the placebo effect and use them, make them work for you.

Mind-body medicine is an umbrella term used for techniques and therapies that take into full consideration the idea that the mind (thoughts and emotions) can influence behavior and health status. Mind-body medicine also considers the influence of a disordered body on thoughts and emotions. The cornucopia of mind-body medical techniques and therapies include, but are not limited to: meditation, hypnotherapy, biofeedback, guided imagery and visualization, yoga, prayer, tai chi, breathing exercises, therapeutic writing and art, music and dance, and perhaps most importantly, cognitive-behavioral therapy. More than two thousand studies in well-respected medical journals give credibility to the value of mind-body medicine. To keep stress in check, improve sleep quality, and maintain a healthy glowing skin, we can choose from a variety of mind-body medicines.

Mindfulness Meditation

The historical use of meditation can be traced back to more than three thousand years ago. Even though different experts have taught numerous variations on the theme of meditation, we can break this technique into two main categories—mindfulness and concentration.

Mindfulness meditation is all about keeping yourself in the "here and now." It is the practice of paying attention to what you are experiencing in the current moment, without drifting off to the worry of the future or the experiences of the past. Mindfulness involves suspending judgment and letting go of opinions so that you will be less reactive. This fosters acceptance, self-reflection, and greater ability to handle difficulties without avoidance.

While the concept of mindfulness is not new, and its values have been discussed for centuries in various traditions, only recently has the scientific world captured the health-promoting potential of mindfulness. In the 1942 textbook *Fundamentals of Medical Dermatology*, many pages are devoted to mindfulness as it relates to sleep and mental rest. The advice cuts to the very heart of the mindfulness-based instructions in every pop self-help book over the past two decades. It is humorous to think that some of the folks who cuddle up with Oprah et al. on talk shows actually think they invented this stuff!

For healthy skin, the textbook advises:

- "Systematic practice at living in the moment and viewing life with serene detachment."
- "Live in the present from one day to the next."
- "Refuse to think of the past, stop speculating, planning, and foreboding for the future."
- "Practice getting outside yourself, viewing your world with detachment, as if looking at it as a parade going by…as a spectator, not a marcher."
- "And one must focus the attention on things that take him (the patient) outside himself. Hence walking out of doors…watching the wind, the clouds, the grass and trees, or if in the city, the life about one, is the proper method."

Remember, this textbook was the basis for what was being taught to young doctors and future dermatologists! This type of wisdom was forgotten when pharmaceutics showed up.

In recent years, mindfulness has been shown to improve inflammatory skin conditions, including dermatitis and psoriasis. Mindfulness almost certainly reduces inflammation by stress-reducing mechanisms. Here are the facts:

- New Japanese research indicates that mindfulness can increase levels of the feel-good chemical serotonin.
- A 2008 study of patients with chronic anxiety shows that instructions on becoming more mindful decreased worry and symptoms of anxiety, which in turn improved sleep quality and daytime energy and mental focus.
- A study in the *Journal of Personality and Social Psychology* (2003) shows that greater awareness and being mindful in life from day to day is correlated with enhanced well-being—improved mood, optimism, life satisfaction, and willingness to attempt new experiences.

Mindfulness of individuals is assessed by inquiring about their focus in the present and preoccupation with past and future. Common questions

include, "Do you snack without being aware that you are eating?" or
"Do you forget someone's name almost immediately after he or she has
told you?"

Structured group programs called mindfulness-based stress reduction
(MBSR) are available at many health institutions. Formal MBSR programs
have been found to be highly effective in lowering stress, decreasing anxiety,
and lifting depression. Some research even indicates that MBSR programs
can insulate and protect against taking on the negative emotions of others
in the workplace.

One study in *Psychosomatic Medicine* (2003) exemplifies the value
of MBSR. Researchers showed that an eight-week mindfulness
course was associated with greater activation of areas of the
brain that govern positive emotions. Even more impressive was that
those who shifted to a greater activation in this positive (happiness,
optimism) area had a better immune response to the flu vaccine.
It is important to note that the beneficial results on mood and the
immune system were not recorded on the day the eight-week
program ended. Instead, the changes were documented four
months after the program's completion.

Breathe Right

One of the most immediate stress busters is simply to focus on the breath.
Meditative breathing, also known as diaphragmatic breathing, is a powerful
and portable technique to have in your stress-reducing arsenal. Many of
us react to stress by over-breathing: our shoulders rise and fall with the
breaths, which is only more likely to push the anxiety cycle. Over-breathing
with short, shallow breaths restricts blood flow to the head and promotes
dizziness, anxiety, fatigue, and other bodily symptoms.

We can change this unhealthy pattern and use breathing as a stress-
reducing ally with a good belly breath. Here we want the abdomen,
and not the upper chest, to do all the moving. To get a handle on this,

place your hand over your belly button, feel it move with your breaths, and imagine a balloon being inflated. You can think of the air flow in abdominal breathing as "in and down" as you develop a natural abdominal movement.

From as far back as 1938, studies have shown that breathing retraining, as it is called, reduces bodily complaints, anxiety levels, and the frequency and intensity of anxiety attacks. Breathing exercises provide a sense of control in dealing with acute and chronic stress. Knowing that at any moment you can use a single, deep belly breath or a few minutes of abdominal breathing reminds us that we can short-circuit the vicious cycle of stress hormones, physiological symptoms, and subsequent interpretation of danger. When you feel less stress overall, your skin will look younger over time. Awareness of breathing can be a great complement to meditation practices, including the concentration meditation we will discuss next.

The Relaxation Response

Concentration meditation, as its name might suggest, involves an intentional and specific focus of cognition. Examples may include an object (such as a picture or candle), a word, phrase, or mantra, or a visualized object. Concentration meditation lifts up our minds and removes us from a mental state of clutter and stress. Everyday hassles of work and commuting, worries on the home front, and day-to-day aggravations are no longer prioritized in the mind of meditation. It is important to note that concentration meditation is a purposeful activity. It is not akin to simply "relaxing" or watching TV.

> Those who regularly practice meditation using a mantra have higher mood levels and sleep-boosting serotonin and melatonin. Their melatonin levels can be as much as 123 percent higher. Both of these chemicals are critical for healthy collagen and skin barrier function. Less stress means younger-looking skin.

The relaxation response is a form of concentration meditation with extensive scientific support. Herbert Benson, MD, of Harvard Medical

School, along with colleagues, was the first to closely examine the physiological effects of transcendental meditation, or the relaxation response. Just as there is a well-defined and automatic stress response (with its associated stress hormones, inflammation, and oxidative stress), so too is there an opposing relaxation response that can be brought on by a form of meditation. The relaxation response promotes deep healing, digestion, and optimal functioning in the body.

Focusing attention on a simple mental stimulus (word, phrase, image) reduces activity of the stress branch of the nervous system. It lowers heart rate, decreases muscle tension, lowers blood pressure, and changes respiratory rate in the opposite direction to hyperventilation. The relaxation response calms down the emotional center of the brain called the limbic system, which in turn reduces stress-related and collagen-destroying hormones such as cortisol. Over time, using the relaxation response provides insulation against daily stressors and enhances resiliency. With practice, it can lower the threat level perceived by stress-prone individuals. This means fewer stress hormones bathing your skin cells.

After years of scientific research, Benson determined that the relaxation response can be initiated by the following:

- A quiet, comfortable environment, with the person in a comfortable position.
- Conscious relaxation of the body's muscles.
- Repetition of a simple mental stimulus such as a word, phrase, image, or prayer.
- A passive mental attitude toward the process itself and any intrusive sounds or thoughts.
- A repetition of the word, phrase, etc. for a duration of 10 to 20 minutes.

Very sophisticated studies are now showing even more value of the relaxation response. For example, brain-wave and MRI studies show that the relaxation response can regulate brain waves associated with relaxed wakefulness, a state of maximal awareness, deep insights, and intuition. The latest study published in the prestigious *PLoS ONE* (2008) journal shows that inducing the relaxation response can influence genetic changes that may be associated with health and longevity.

YOGA, TAI CHI, AND QI GONG

Yoga, tai chi, and its cousin qi gong bring together physical movement and the emotional being, a union that epitomizes mind-body medicine. Among Westerners, Hatha yoga has become the most popular form. Hatha (physical) yoga incorporates specific movements and postures (asana), and breathing techniques (pranayama) often used along with meditation. In Hatha yoga, the breath takes center stage. Through proper breathing control, one can absorb the life force, or prana. The breath is the essential component in the union of mind and body. After three months of practice, yoga boosts melatonin levels and overall well-being. It can also improve sleep and reduce the perception of stress.

Researchers from Bangalore, India, showed that regular practice of yoga may be akin to a sleeping pill. In adults with insomnia, those practicing yoga reduced the time it takes to get to sleep down from 40 minutes to 10 minutes. Yoga practice also added an hour on to total sleep time.

In the *Annals of Behavioral Medicine* (2004), researchers showed that Hatha yoga can reduce cortisol levels and improve scores on the Perceived Stress Scale.

In 2007, researchers from Harvard showed that yoga sessions can boost GABA levels in the brain by 27 percent, providing a physiological mechanism for yoga's ability to lower stress and anxiety.

Qi gong and tai chi also combine physical movement, breathing, and meditation, which can promote the relaxation response and improve mental clarity. The focused breathing and movement are said to enhance the flow of energy (qi, pronounced "chee") throughout the body. Regular practice of tai chi improves cardiovascular and lung function, strength, balance, flexibility, blood flow, and psychological parameters. As with yoga, tai chi and qi gong can reduce collagen-disrupting cortisol. In a year-long study published in the *Journal of Physical Activity and Health* (2009), researchers showed that regular participation in tai chi not only lowered oxidative stress, but also reduced glycation and protected against DNA damage.

Exercise

Beyond yoga and tai chi, exercise is an effective tool in stress reduction and improving mental outlook. Indeed, the strength of exercise as a medical intervention can actually extend into the psychiatrist's office. It has been shown to be a viable means of treating depression and anxiety disorders. Exercise appears to provide a resiliency against stress and improve sleep. Overall physical fitness is also associated with lower levels of inflammatory chemicals circulating around the body.

Of particular relevance to maintaining youthful skin: exercise in older adults can prevent the age-related decline in blood flow to the far reaches of the skin. Note, you do not have to exercise to the point of exhaustion. Simply walking may be one of the most important ways to maintain cardiovascular health and stave off cognitive decline with aging. The authors of the 1942 dermatology textbook said it best: "While there are many elaborate and expensive devices for discharge of tension...just plain walking remains the simplest, cheapest, and most effective of them all."

Cognitive-Behavioral Appraisal

Quite obviously, negative thinking feeds the stress cycle and promotes poor lifestyle, or behavioral choices. Therefore, cognitions, or thoughts, can have a negative impact on behavior. In turn, inappropriate and health-compromising behaviors can influence our thoughts in a vicious cycle. Cognitive-behavioral appraisal (CBA) can cut off this process. CBA is well known to be helpful for anxiety, depression, and other chronic illnesses. As a therapy, CBA is not limited to very ill people. It can also be used to promote and maintain overall health and keep stress in check.

One goal of CBA is to identify and address negative thoughts and beliefs. Through CBA, we can identify the so-called cognitive distortions that eliminate the positive, over-exaggerate the negative, and invoke a lot of "What if?" future thinking. These thoughts are almost always "What if..." plus a negative. For example, "What if I do poorly on the test?" "What if I forget my lines?" "What if my presentation is not well received?" "What if that stomachache is cancer?" "What if the elevator gets stuck?"... and on it goes.

Sometimes stressed individuals take those thoughts to the next level: the failed test means that the individual will never get a decent job and will never be successful; the elevator that gets stuck will mean missing the meeting and losing the important business deal. Our "what ifs" usually feed into more catastrophic thinking, which, in turn, feeds the stress chemicals. Remember, when you think it, you can start to *believe* it, and your body will respond as if the stress is actually happening.

More fuel on the stress fire comes from leaping to conclusions. To cut off the stress cycle, it is important not to draw firm conclusions before the facts are in. Reshaping thoughts and beliefs, underscoring the positive "what ifs" and staying in the moment can minimize stress and enhance coping skills.

CBA can help identify self-imposed pressures and the internal talk that generates stress. Quite often, individuals who are prone to stress place a tremendous amount of pressure on themselves and are unable to say no to burdensome obligations. The authors of the 1942 dermatology textbook recognized that the burden of "must do" was a primary cause of stress. They urged dermatologists of the day to educate patients that there were alternatives, recommending: "Sift out essential from nonessential obligations—you will think them all essential at first—and reject, turn down, back out of 50–90 percent of the nonessentials. For the time being, anything that says 'you must' to you should be answered with a flat refusal. Don't do 'you musts.'"

Most of the negatives identified in CBA are related to aspects of self-talk. Our inner dialog influences our feelings, and positive self-talk generates positive feelings. Inner dialog is one of the few things that we can control. Thinking "I am competent and I can cope with this" is clearly a better option than "There is no way I can do this." Thinking, "What if my presentation goes great?" is definitely better than "What if the presentation is too much for me to handle?" Thinking and believing that you are calm, in a relaxed state, and in control of your breathing is much more likely to give you an actual sense of control. With practice, learning to direct self-talk will help to keep you in the here and now, ultimately reducing stress and generating a new reality.

The insights of CBA help to foster self-acceptance, the understanding that we don't have to be a super-hero in daily life. As stated by John Stokes et al. in 1942, "Accept yourself as you are, not as you think you might, ought, or would like to be. Self-acceptance, limitations and all, is the beginning of contentment, which is tension release and rest for the nervous system." CBA has great potential to improve your daily quality of life, ultimately turning down the dial on the collagen and skin-barrier-disrupting inflammation and oxidative stress.

COGNITIVE DISTORTIONS

- All-or-nothing thinking: Things are either good or bad; there is no middle ground.
- Overgeneralization: Stress-prone individuals may view negative events as a continuous pattern of defeat.
- Filter out positives: Stress-prone individuals may filter the world with glasses that ignore the positive and let the negative events gain access to the brain. Accomplishments are discounted and not used to enhance coping for future events.
- Jumping to conclusions: Stress-prone individuals make rapid conclusions in the absence of solid evidence. For example, the headache is a brain tumor. Turbulence is mechanical difficulties or an incompetent pilot on a plane.
- Mind reading: Getting into others' heads and assuming that people are reacting negatively to you.
- Fortune-telling: Even with no crystal ball, predicting that things will turn out badly.
- Magnification: Stress-prone individuals may consider events or challenges to be much more challenging than they really are.
- Emotional reasoning: You reason from how you feel—"I feel incompetent, so I must actually be incompetent."

- "Should" statements: Stress-prone individuals may criticize themselves or others with definitive "shoulds," "shouldn'ts," "musts," "oughts," and "have-tos."
- Labeling: Everyone makes mistakes and struggles. However, the stress-hardy individual will say "I made a mistake," but the stress-prone will say, "I am not a strong person" or "I am so incompetent."
- Blame: Stress-prone individuals may blame themselves for something they were not entirely responsible for, or may blame others.

Jump into Nature

North Americans may be going green with exciting environmental initiatives, yet in reality we are turning our backs on nature. Nature-based recreation has been on the decline since the late 1980s and early 1990s. Visits to state and national parks in the United States have been on a steady decline over the past two decades. The same phenomenon is occurring in Japan. The reason is not due to a decline in the attractiveness of public parks. It is linked to our infatuation with video games and computers. In the battle for your recreation time, Best Buy has won out over coniferous trees and waterfalls.

This is a sorry state of affairs, considering the health implications. Natural environments, particularly green forested areas, have stress-reducing power. As proposed by environmental psychologist Stephen Kaplan, PhD, the reason we feel so refreshed after time spent in natural settings is that, in nature, little effort is required to inhibit unwanted stimuli. In indoor settings, such as sitting in front of computer screens in a busy office or shopping in a crowded, noisy mall, you must constantly and deliberately direct attention to the task at hand because of a multitude of unwanted stimuli.

Seeing green appears to ground us from overload and may even improve cognition and reduce impulsive behavior. The air in natural environments—including at the beach, near waterfalls, and within forests, among others—is much higher in negative ions. Negative air ions are known to influence mood in a generally positive way: they promote our antioxidant defense system, lower blood lactate, and improve aerobic metabolism via enhancing blood flow.

Negative air ions are natural components of surrounding and exhaled air. So they are much higher in natural settings, after rain, near oceans and waterfalls, and inside woodlands. Negative ions are depleted within polluted, enclosed, and air-conditioned rooms. So they are not in abundance in homes and offices, and they are depleted by electronic devices, particularly computer screens and televisions.

In Japan, the practice of forest-air bathing is called *shinrin-yoku*, and it has been used medicinally for many years. In a study published in the *International Journal of Biometeorology* (1998), researchers from the Hokkaido School of Medicine showed that walking in forest air lowers the stress hormone cortisol, decreases glycation, and improves well-being.

Two separate studies in the *Journal of Physiological Anthropology* (2007) showed that *shinrin-yoku*, exercising in the forest, reduced activity in areas of the brain associated with stress, lowered cortisol, and reduced overall stress, as compared to a similar amount of exercise in a city environment.

The effects of woodland walking, therefore, appear to be above and beyond the value of exercise alone. The authors attribute some of the benefits to the volatile compounds within the forest air. Bathing your skin in forest air may be a very effective way to limit internal effects against your collagen.

Do your best to see green and expose yourself to natural settings. Every little bit helps: even the addition of plants to a workplace has been shown to reduce physiological responses to stress, and merely having a window view in a hospital is associated with overall recovery from surgery and significantly less use of pain medication.

Scents of Relaxation

Scientific evaluation of aromatherapy is finally being approached with some degree of sophistication. This is highlighted by a recent study in *Neuroscience Letters* (2008) that showed aromatherapy can lower activity in the area of the brain associated with stress and decrease the production of excess sebum (oil) in stressed adults. The beneficial effects of certain aromas on the mental outlook of humans have been touted for centuries, and most of us are aware that simply talking about an aroma can bring up memories of the past. The human olfactory system is intricately tied to the limbic system, the area of the brain that is a busy hub and the control center of emotional communication.

A number of recent studies have shown that essential oils can reduce stress, promote relaxation, and enhance cognitive function. Based on the research, we can make some generalizations about aromas. For example, lavender and rosemary may lower cortisol in adults under stress. However, stress reduction in the real world depends on the oil itself and personal preferences. For example, Japanese researchers showed that jasmine can reduce experimental stress in most young adults who volunteered for a study. But jasmine increased anxiety in those who said before the experiment that they did not like that floral smell.

Based on your personal preferences, you might try one of these:

- Improve positive emotions with the smell of lemon oil.
- Reduce daytime sleepiness with peppermint oil.
- Promote sleep quality and increase alertness the following day with jasmine.
- Reduce road rage with peppermint and cinnamon.

THIS IS YOUR BRAIN ON AROMAS

In an interesting study from Wheeling Jesuit University, researchers looked at the effects of jasmine, lavender, or no scent for three nights. The aromatherapy was infused into the rooms at such low levels that many sleepers were not even aware of any aroma at all.

Not only did the jasmine sleepers toss and turn less frequently, but they woke up feeling less anxiety the next day. The jasmine sleepers also performed better on cognitive testing the next day. Lavender was good, too, but it couldn't match the effects of jasmine.

The same group from Wheeling recently showed that peppermint and cinnamon aromatherapy may quell road rage. They showed that prolonged driving led to the expected increased anger, fatigue, and physical demand, as well as decreased energy. Peppermint and cinnamon both decreased driving frustration and increased alertness while driving. Interestingly, the aroma of fast food made things worse! Peppermint was specifically shown to lower levels of anxiety related to the extended driving. Keep a bottle of your favorite aromatherapy on hand in the center console of your car. You never know when you may need it.

Writing and Journaling

For centuries, human beings have expressed themselves emotionally in writing and art. Confronting difficult life experiences through writing and art can have very positive effects on both emotional and physical well-being. Although writing about traumatic or particularly difficult life events can be difficult at the time, it leads to subsequent mood elevation and decreased use of healthcare services. Dozens of studies show that writing about stressful or traumatic events can improve various health conditions or well-being, or both.

Taking advantage of therapeutic writing involves the expression of deeply held emotions, including what you feel and why you feel it. Although you may want to share your writings, it is best to write just for yourself and with the intention of destroying the writing. If you set out with the mindset that you will shred the material, you will be less likely to hold back. If events are constantly on your mind, this may be time to write things down or draw them out. Using pen and paper may be better than typing on a computer; one study showed that typing about difficult life events evokes less emotional arousal and less self-disclosure than writing it out old-school style with longhand. Writing and artwork related to serious traumatic events would be best conducted with guidance from a mental health professional.

The Three Cs

Some folks never seem to get stressed out no matter what. All hell can break loose, and it just doesn't seem to faze them. Rather than being jealous of these individuals, it may be worthwhile to see how we can learn from them. There are three defining and consistent characteristics of adults with so-called stress-hardiness—people who seem resilient to stress and its consequences.

> Challenge, control, and commitment are the three Cs that stress-hardy people embrace in their daily outlook.

Stress-hardy individuals view change as a challenge rather than something to be feared. People who are prone to stress detest change, while the stress-hardy view it as a normal part of life, something that represents a stimulus for growth and maturity rather than a threat.

With regard to control, hardy personalities believe their actions make a difference. They believe that they have control and are not merely a victim of fate. In most cases, stress-hardy individuals have no more control over events than those who are stress-prone…they just believe they do.

Finally, stress-hardy individuals are immersed in what they do in life. They are committed to the end, stick with the task at hand, and problem solve it out, all the while remaining truly engaged in life, instead of focusing simply on getting from Point A to Point B.

The Best for Last

Thinking about the realities of stress can be overwhelming: it's easy to get wrapped up in the doom and gloom. Yes, chronic stress can impact overall health, longevity, and certainly the visible signs of aging. However, as we've reviewed, lots of different ways can be used to keep stress managed and in check. Our discussion is obviously not an exhaustive one, although

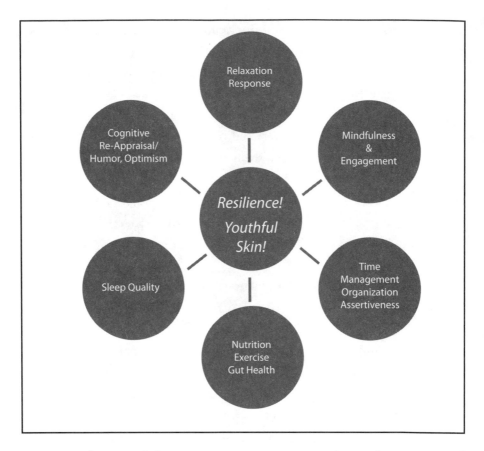

we covered some of the primary interventions used to reduce stress and improve sleep quality. Some other general considerations include, but are not limited to: organizational skills, time management, prioritizing tasks and life goals, delegating, letting go of procrastination, using humor, being optimistic, and taking advantage of social support.

Researchers from the University of California, San Francisco, published a landmark study in the journal *Lancet Oncology* (2008) that should fill all of us with hope. Here we have saved the best for last. A team of cutting-edge physicians and scientists showed in humans, not lab mice, that a three-month lifestyle intervention improved the activity of the enzymes that protect your telomeres (protective caps at the end of DNA). A healthy diet rich in fruits, vegetables, whole grains, legumes, and soy—combined with an exercise and stress management intervention and four dietary supplements (fish oil, selenium, and vitamins C and E)—improved telomerase activity.

Simply put, here's the hopeful finding: telomerase activity, the enzyme of longevity, is decreased with stress, decreased with inflammation, decreased with oxidative stress, and decreased with cortisol. This decline of activity is, in turn, associated with accelerated aging. *A lifestyle intervention with diet and stress management increases telomerase activity not just a little, but by 30 percent!* This is one of the most important studies of our time.

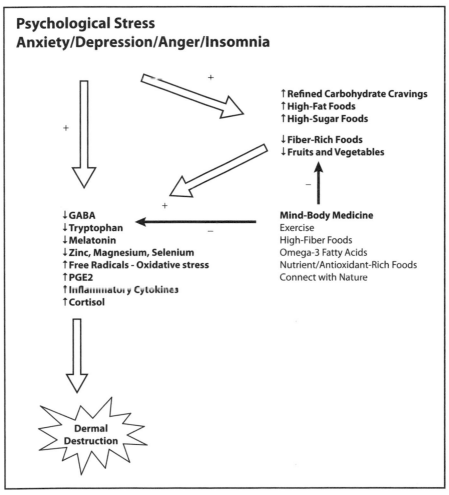

Psychological Stress
Anxiety/Depression/Anger/Insomnia

↑ **Refined Carbohydrate Cravings**
↑ **High-Fat Foods**
↑ **High-Sugar Foods**

↓ **Fiber-Rich Foods**
↓ **Fruits and Vegetables**

↓ **GABA**
↓ **Tryptophan**
↓ **Melatonin**
↓ **Zinc, Magnesium, Selenium**
↑ **Free Radicals - Oxidative stress**
↑ **PGE2**
↑ **Inflammatory Cytokines**
↑ **Cortisol**

Mind-Body Medicine
Exercise
High-Fiber Foods
Omega-3 Fatty Acids
Nutrient/Antioxidant-Rich Foods
Connect with Nature

Dermal Destruction

Summary: Psychological stress and insomnia directly promote (+) the production of collagen-destroying free radicals and inflammatory chemicals. Stress also depletes collagen-protecting GABA, tryptophan, melatonin and skin anti-aging nutrients. An indirect influence is also apparent via changing dietary choices. Stress management, exercise and nutrient-dense foods cut off (–) the skin aging cycle by lowering inflammation and oxidative stress and restoring the collagen-protecting nutrients and chemicals.

Skin Food I:
Dietary Supplements

THE USE OF NUTRITIONAL AND HERBAL products by North Americans has never been higher. Long gone are the days when a select few vitamins and minerals were the only choices in the drugstore. Today, Americans spend more than 25 billion dollars annually on dietary supplements, and at last count, there were more than 29,000 different commercially available supplements. North Americans generally use dietary supplements for three main reasons—to enhance dietary quality, as a preventive influence against disease, and as a "natural" way to address health problems. Among the preventive and health-promoting reasons for consuming supplements, many adults report benefits to the skin.

The sometimes murky waters of dietary supplements can be a sea of confusion for consumers. More than 40 percent of average American and Canadian adults take at least one dietary supplement on a regular basis. Researchers from the University of California, Los Angeles, found that patients in consultation for cosmetic surgery were twice as likely as the general population to be taking some sort of dietary supplement.

While many adults take supplements to improve the skin's appearance, studies indicate that consumers are unsure how and why an internal product might help the skin. We will guide you through the marketing and media hype, pare down the need to take bags and bags of supplements, and provide a research-based appraisal to support our top supplement picks.

History of Dietary Supplements

While the dizzying array of products formulated to promote beauty from the inside may be new, and the catchy names for the concept—skingestibles or nutricosmetics—may be additions to the contemporary lexicon, the idea itself is not new. The press releases would have us believe that the folks who thought of putting vitamins in water for the promotion of beauty had done something akin to splitting the atom. In truth, the use of oral nutritional supplements to enhance beauty from the inside dates back almost to the discovery of vitamins in food.

Vitamin A supplements have been used to improve facial appearance and reduce acne for about eighty years. Supplements with B vitamins, particularly yeast (brewer's and other forms of medicinal yeast rich in B vitamins), have been touted for improving the appearance of the skin since the early 1920s. In fact, early B-vitamin skin supplements were actually individually wrapped yeast cakes to be consumed on a regular basis! Studies in the 1930s and 1940s suggested that vitamin C and some of the B vitamins may have anti-aging properties, and so-called skin vitamin formulas appeared on the market. Scientists had shown that vitamins are found in the skin in higher amounts than previously thought, particularly vitamin C and the B vitamin niacin.

A sprinkling of older studies showed that vitamin supplements could have some value in improving inflammatory skin conditions. However, with the advent of powerful drugs and topical preparations in the 1950s, the interest and enthusiasm for internal beauty supplements waned. Even where interest continued in vitamins and fats as skin-related supplements, it was almost exclusively in the topical domain. Beyond meeting the minimal recommended dietary allowance (RDA), nutritional supplements were largely a non-issue in the dermatological arsenal.

In the 1970s, there was not only disinterest in dietary supplements, but also almost complete resistance to them in the dermatological community. The prevailing notion was that health food and supplements were a waste, and that North Americans should basically eat whatever mass-market

"Now my skin's as smooth as satin"

"No more skin blemishes. I've taken three bottles of Yeast Foam Tablets and for the first time in months my skin now is smooth as satin." Yeast Foam Tablets correct skin ailments in the *natural* way —by reaching the root of the trouble and supplying the system with an element necessary to a correct diet and good health.

Made of whole, selected yeast. Easy to take; they keep and they don't cause gas. Unexcelled for appetite and digestion troubles. For adults and children, too. Sold by all druggists.

Made by the makers of Yeast Foam and Magic Yeast

Yeast Foam Tablets
A Tonic Food

Send for large free sample—Yeast Foam Tablets

*Your name*_____

*Address*_____

Mail coupon to Northwestern Yeast Company
1750 North Ashland Avenue, Chicago   LD-3-24

So you thought skingestibles were new? B vitamin tablets from yeast are promoted for smooth, glowing skin in 1924.

corporations provided. One dermatologist summed up the attitude in the *American Family Physician* journal (1971): "...too many patients harbor the delusion that their health can somehow be mysteriously harmed by something in their diet."

The Comeback

Fast-forward to 2009, and we see massive changes. Results of the Healthcare Professionals Impact Study (January 2009) showed that most dermatologists now view dietary supplements in a favorable light. Specifically, two thirds of a sample of three hundred American dermatologists recommended dietary supplements to their patients. The top reason cited for doing so was primarily for the support of healthy skin. More than 60 percent of the dermatologists reported nutritional gaps in the diet of the average patient, and their belief that dietary supplements might help address such voids. On the whole, 71 percent of dermatologists reported that a healthy diet, vitamins, and other supplements—along with exercise and healthy lifestyle choices—are of importance to healthy skin.

So what happened along the way to change attitudes from complete disdain to acceptance of supplements? Why are most dermatologists frequently asked about dietary supplements, particularly vitamins C, D, and E and fish oil? How did we go from the basic "skin vitamin" messages of the 1930s and 1940s to a nutricosmetic industry of skin-based oral supplements that is said to be valued at 3 billion dollars annually?

The comeback of internal beauty supplements occurred via a perfect storm in the early 1990s. During this time, a constellation of events renewed interest in the potential value of supplements. First came studies showing that dietary supplements, including antioxidant vitamins C and E, as well as fish oil, might help protect against damage from UV radiation. We also had *Time* magazine making vitamins the cover story on April 6, 1992, along with a tagline indicating that vitamins might halt the "ravages of aging." In addition, university-based research and corporate involvement began to reach a new degree of sophistication, and things were looking rosy for a business fueled by the first boomers, who were turning forty-six.

Still, most mainstream skin specialists dismissed studies pertaining to UV protection as only low-impact news. The general thinking was that the results might translate into useful advances in topical preparations, but they would not be a catalyst in driving the immediate sales of fish oil and multivitamins for skin health. Protecting against UV damage from the inside seemed like a long-term investment. Any revival of internal skin supplements had to be based on real results that were relatively immediate, taking place in sixty to ninety days. As part of the perfect storm, researchers from Finland would highlight the more rapid anti-aging value of oral fish collagen supplements in 1991 and 1992, and the nutricosmetic industry was reborn.

Fish Collagen and GAGs

Oral supplementation with marine-fish cartilage (with collagen and glycosaminoglycans, or GAGs) can significantly improve the appearance of the skin. Dermal thickness increases, and overall elasticity is significantly improved. Fish collagen, or more specifically, hydrolyzed (meaning "water-broken" or "water-digested") fish collagen is a major staple of anti-aging, internal beauty. When first discovered, the sales of oral collagen for skin took off like wildfire in Japan.

Still, it seemed implausible: how on earth could oral fish collagen and GAGs influence the skin? Isn't fish collagen degraded into individual amino acids in the digestive tract, just like any other protein? Don't enzymes in the blood break down any intact linkages of small amino-acid groups (peptides)? Such were the questions of the skeptic and naysayer.

But fish collagen works. Small peptide units, including some of those from orally ingested collagen, are absorbed intact through the intestinal passages. Some of the peptides of collagen are resistant to breakdown by enzymes in the blood. Peptides of oral collagen can act as a signal to turn on fibroblast activity and even provide antioxidant support in the skin. The true benefit of fish cartilage, though, is that it reduces fine lines and dryness, and improves skin tone, providing a more even color distribution of the skin. Once again, visible benefits are backed up by increased dermal thickness, less wrinkling, and improved elasticity.

Two different studies in 2004 showed that fish peptides can make a difference in hydration. The first, a German study from the University of Witten, showed a significant reduction in water loss from the skin after three months of supplementation. The second, a Japanese study in the *Journal of Nutritional Food* (2004), showed that oral consumption of hydrolyzed collagen for two months could improve hydration in adult women.

The latest research trend with marine-fish peptides is to combine them with antioxidants and other skin-supporting ingredients. A 2005 study showed that oral consumption of 700 milligrams of a fish peptide daily—along with 200 milligrams of alpha-lipoic acid, 180 milligrams of vitamin C, 24 milligrams of zinc, 4 milligrams of lycopene, and some B vitamins—improved skin thickness, elasticity, and self-evaluations of the visible signs of aging. Positive results were noticed after two months of use.

In a study published in the *European Journal of Clinical Nutrition* (2006), researchers from the University of Copenhagen reported the value of a fish protein extract—along with 350 milligrams of soy extract and some lycopene and white tea extract— compared to placebo. In this case, six months of use resulted in a significant reduction in forehead and eye wrinkles, as well as overall sagging and laxity of the skin. The researchers backed up the clinical and photographically judged improvements with objective ultrasound measurements showing improved dermal density, as compared with those in the placebo group. Anti-oxidants, it seems, can enhance the role of fish-collagen extracts in skin-care supplementation.

GLUCOSAMINE—NOT JUST FOR YOUR JOINTS

One of the most popular dietary supplements in North America, best known for its ability to reduce osteoarthritis, is glucosamine. Oral supplementation with glucosamine can reduce inflammation in the joint and provide the raw materials for repair of cartilage through the aging process. Since glucosamine can also provide the raw materials to build glycosaminoglycans (GAGs, the important dermal structural components), its potential for aging skin has not been lost on cosmetic dermatologists.

A study published in the *Journal of Cosmetic Science* (2006) high-lighted the ability of a skin-friendly form of glucosamine—N-acetyl glucosamine—to improve the appearance of aging skin. Specifically, 1,000 milligrams of oral glucosamine improved hydration of the skin, and a topical preparation of 2 percent glucosamine improved facial wrinkles, particularly those around the eyes. Look for glucosamine as an emerging star ingredient in oral and topical skin supplements.

Antioxidants

As previously discussed, oral antioxidants make it to the far reaches of the skin layers, but do they actually make a clinical difference? Is it all about future protection against the ravages of aging, or are there more immediate benefits to the appearance of the skin?

The answer is yes, there are immediate benefits, which are real-world results showing relatively fast improvements in overall texture, tone, and hydration of the skin. In fact, the result can be more glowing and well-hydrated skin within twenty-one days. In a study published in the *International Journal of Cosmetic Science* (2002), Italian researchers reported that oral ingestion of a mixture of carotenoid antioxidants (6 milligrams of lutein and 0.3 milligrams of zeaxanthin daily) could improve hydration and skin-barrier function by increasing the lipids in the outer layers of the skin.

A unique finding, it suggested that antioxidants are not just protecting collagen—but also intricately involved in fat regulation in the skin. The study underscores a theme within nutritional medicine: all things nutritional are intertwined in the body. Looking at the results from a distance, it would seem implausible that oral antioxidant supplements could influence skin-barrier lipids, but influence they do.

More recently a joint U.S. and European study published in *Skin Pharmacology and Physiology* (2007) found that 10 milligrams of lutein and 0.6 milligrams of zeaxanthin per day do indeed increase skin lipids, improve elasticity, and improve hydration in adults. The beneficial influence of these oral carotenoid antioxidants on the appearance of skin was multiplied when a topical preparation with carotenoid antioxidants was combined with the oral supplements. This would support our own stance in addressing the visible signs of aging from a nutritional perspective—feed the skin internally and externally.

In a landmark study published in *Skin Pharmacology and Physiology* (2006), German investigators found significant reductions in roughness, scaling, and wrinkling of the skin in those consuming an oral mix of lycopene, selenium, vitamin E, beta-carotene, and lutein. Ultrasound measurements showed the antioxidants had a significant influence in increasing dermal thickness, and a scanning device showed the skin to be smoother. Almost certainly, the synergy of the antioxidants is the central reason for the beneficial results.

> **Added-Value Multivitamin Formulas:** Since experts recommend that all North American's take a daily multivitamin, and many adults concerned about skin health also take additional supplements, a few companies are now making skin-specific multivitamin formulas. Typically these are full-spectrum multivitamin and mineral formulas with added ingredients such as fish collagen, antioxidants from lycopene, fruits, berry, and tea extracts. One such commercially available multivitamin is multi+ daily glow from Genuine Health.

Essential Fats

Over time, the anti-inflammatory and UV-protecting properties of omega-3 fatty acids and gamma-linolenic acid (GLA) from borage oil unquestionably minimize the aging process.

A combination of oral omega-3 from fish oil and GLA was recently investigated in healthy women aged forty to sixty. The intervention used just over 1 gram of EPA from fish oil, along with smaller amounts of DHA and GLA, taken daily for three months. While the supplement made no difference at the six-week mark, there was significant improvement in the elasticity of the skin between the six- and twelve-week assessments. The study also showed trends toward an improvement in epidermal-barrier function with the supplement use.

While a number of studies have shown the value of essential fatty acids in inflammatory skin disorders, these emerging studies in healthy adults show that fish oil and borage oil should be a central part of basic skin care. Remember, we cannot make these fats. We are completely reliant upon dietary intake.

SKIN ANTI-AGING NUTRIENT HIGHLIGHT: ZINC

What is it?

Zinc is an essential mineral involved in more than three hundred different enzyme reactions, so not surprisingly, zinc has a hand in many biological systems within the body. Zinc's important role has been documented in growth and development, brain function, immune function, and reproduction, to name a few. Zinc can be found in oysters, lean meats, beans, nuts, seeds oatmeal, whole grains, and Japanese miso.

Why is it of value?

Zinc is one of the most important antioxidant and anti-inflamma-tory nutrients for the support of glowing skin. Zinc has been shown to protect against damage from UV radiation and to exert anti-aging properties in the face of environmental assault. Zinc and selenium support the fibroblasts, the cells that make collagen. Zinc is also involved in the metabolism of omega-3 fatty acids, and emerging studies show that zinc may be of value in protecting against depression.

Probiotics

Probiotics are the friendly, viable bacteria that have the potential to positively influence health. As we reviewed in chapter 4, the value of beneficial bacteria inside the intestines may have far-reaching effects way beyond the gut. In fact, the microbes of the intestinal tract may influence nerve-cell communication and even human behavior. We have come a long way from the early days of *Lactobacillus* research, and new encapsulation techniques allow for shelf-stable strains of beneficial bacteria.

Two recent studies highlight the importance of probiotics in relation to the absorption of other skin-friendly nutrients and essential fats. The first showed that oral collagen administered in the form of a *Lactobacillus* yogurt drink significantly increased the collagen-building proteins in the bloodstream. The second showed that a probiotic yogurt drink with green tea, borage oil, and vitamin E significantly improved barrier function of the stratum corneum versus placebo (non-probiotic acidified milk) after six weeks.

Administering the probiotics and the GLA together seemed to improve the absorption of the GLA: the total amount of GLA making it to the bloodstream doubled during the study! Of course, it is impossible to say that the probiotics alone improved the skin barrier and hydration. The green tea, the GLA, the vitamin E, or some combination of the three may have been responsible. The point is that taking probiotic supplements may be of value for many reasons, including the enhanced absorption of collagen peptides and the other anti-aging ingredients found in dietary supplements.

The big question surrounding probiotics is which supplement or yogurt should be recommended for the maintenance of youthful skin. Many probiotic formulas are on the market, so finding a brand with therapeutic levels of viable bacteria inside the bottle or the yogurt container can be a challenge. There are few, if any, live bacteria in commercial pills, powders, and yogurts.

A *Consumer Reports* exposé in 2005 highlighted many problems with probiotic yogurts and pills. Most experts agree that one billion colony-forming units (CFUs) of bacteria is the minimal level needed to produce meaningful benefits. The researchers at *Consumer Reports* found that probiotic formulas quite often fell short in CFUs.

In addition, the beneficial effects of probiotics appear to be very much related to the strain of bacteria involved. Sadly, probiotics are still marketed under the umbrella term *acidophilus*, leading consumers to believe that any old probiotic (or acidophilus!) will do. Such is obviously not the case, and you should know the three important parts to any probiotic name—genus, species, and strain. For example, two of the more researched strains in the world are *Lactobacillus* (genus) *casei* (species) Shirota (strain) and

Lactobacillus (genus) *plantarum* (species) 299V (strain). These are well-documented bacterial strains that have been the subject of scientific and medical research.

We believe that probiotics are an essential part of the nutritional approaches to keeping your skin younger and we have placed our most trusted recommendations for probiotics and yogurts in the appendices.

Combination Supplements

Given that oral antioxidants, essential fatty acids, vitamins, and fish collagen can all contribute to the maintenance of youthful skin, it shouldn't come as a big surprise that researchers have been looking at food supplements that contain all of these ingredients. In general, combination supplements with these ingredients work wonders for your skin, keeping it well-hydrated and supple, with a decrease in facial furrows.

One study involved a food supplement with undisclosed amounts of fish oil, borage oil, lycopene, vitamin E, rice extract with vegetable ceramides, and marine peptides from fish cartilage. Remember the ceramides? These are fats that make up the mortar between the bricks of your epidermal skin barrier. Ceramides occur in plants, especially rice. After forty days on the combination food supplement (vs. placebo), individuals had smoother skin, and epidermal barrier function improved, keeping water loss in check. Skin roughness improved by 25 percent, and dryness decreased by almost 60 percent. Perhaps most impressive was the 24 percent reduction in the volume of facial furrows.

The second investigation of a combination food supplement for changes to skin appearance evaluated the potential value of a daily food supplement containing fish and borage oils (about 1 gram), green tea extract (400 milligrams), grape extract (150 milligrams), marine cartilage (100 milligrams), and smaller amounts of B vitamins, along with selenium, chromium, and beta-carotene. A total of fifty-two middle-aged women consumed the nutrient combination for about two months, after which they were evaluated for skin hydration, wrinkles, and skin surface creasing.

After the fifty-six-day supplement intervention, wrinkle depth decreased by more than 27 percent, and wrinkle volume decreased by almost 23 percent. In addition, overall skin hydration improved significantly. The results highlight the potential value of food-based supplements, including the so-called super-food category of powdered green foods and dehydrated mixes of berries, herbs, fruits, and vegetables. Look for products with added ingredients specific for skin, such as cocoa extracts and fish collagen.

SKIN ANTI-AGING NUTRIENT HIGHLIGHT: SELENIUM

What is it?
Selenium is a minor mineral that pulls quite a bit of weight in the body. Selenium is required for the function of many enzymes throughout the body, including those involved in the immune and antioxidant defense systems. Sources include whole grains, nuts, seafood, salmon, and halibut.

Why is it of value?
Selenium is critical to the workings of the antioxidant system within the skin. It allows one of the most important antioxidants in the human body, glutathione, to do its job. Selenium has been shown to work synergistically with, and to preserve the levels of, other antioxidants. The selenium-dependent enzyme that controls glutathione is low in patients with chronic skin conditions and works overtime when the skin is faced with environmental assaults. Research has shown that selenium may protect against damage from UV radiation and also may work synergistically with zinc to protect against UV-induced skin aging.

Super-Food Category

Walk into any decent health-food store, and you will notice an ever-expanding section known as super-foods. The availability of whole fruit, vegetable, and herbal extracts in powder form is an exciting development in the supplement world. Modern extraction techniques remove the water from fruits, vegetables, and herbs while leaving the nutrients behind. This means you can add specific skin-saving nutrients to a variety of your own foods and beverages.

> The Japanese popularized powdered, green-and-purple food supplements and the technical advances that allowed for their development. In 1969, the first powdered "*aojiru*" (a powdered combination of dehydrated kale and barley grass) was introduced to the masses. More recently, research has supported the use of food-based blends, including a super-food from Genuine Health of Canada. In this case, researchers from the University of Toronto reported in the *Canadian Journal of Dietetic Practice and Research* (2004) that this unique blend of foods and herbs can improve energy levels in healthy, but tired women.
>
> The study involved more than one hundred otherwise healthy women from Toronto, Canada, who consumed the super-food (greens+) or a carefully matched (placebo) powdered beverage for three months. Subjects were evaluated using various validated questionnaires. Those taking the actual super-food were found to have improvements in vitality and had significantly more energy than those in the placebo group. (See the Appendices for details on Genuine Health.)

Most super-food supplements contain a broad array of powdered ingredients, including berries, exotic fruits, the Brassica family vegetables, cocoa, turmeric, ginger, cinnamon, green leafy vegetables, beets, apple skins, sprouts, and whole grains such as brown rice.

> The bottom line is that many of the ingredients in super-food supplements are the very ones that promote youthful skin.

These products allow for the consistent intake of low to moderate levels of antioxidant-rich plants. In contrast to isolated antioxidants (for example, vitamin C or E alone), these supplements are better suited to provide the advantage of whole foods—the synergy factor. A good super-food product will avoid mega-doses of any particular ingredient; instead, it should supply a colorful blend of the much-needed phytochemicals and nutrients that are obviously absent from the average North American diet.

To be clear, we are not suggesting that super-food supplements are a substitute for a plate full of colorful fruits and vegetables. They are, however, a good insurance policy to ensure adequate intake of a variety of skin-defending phytochemicals. One of the reasons that we are supportive of super-food formulas is that they help to put a big dent in the top-heavy acid load in the North American diet. Our overconsumption of acid-heavy meats, dairy, and processed grains is not without consequence to the aging process and the appearance of our skin. Let's explore the pH story in more detail.

COCOA, COSMECEUTICALS, AND CANDY

Are the exciting new studies showing that 329 milligrams of cocoa antioxidants improve blood flow to the skin, increase hydration, and decrease roughness and scaling of the skin in otherwise healthy middle-aged women an excuse to binge on chocolate?

The excitement of the research studies should be tempered with the reality that, depending on brand, about 40 grams or more of dark chocolate (70 percent cocoa) would be needed to attain the levels of antioxidants used in the study. This translates into 15 grams of fat, 12 grams of sugar, and somewhere in the range of 250 calories. If you tried to get to the 329 milligrams of cocoa antioxidants from mass-marketed hot cocoa, you would need to drink 3.5 servings. Even mixed with 2 percent low-fat milk, that would cost you 700 calories, 84 grams of sugar, and 28 grams of fat.

One alternative would be the cosmeceutical delivery of the 329 milligrams of cocoa antioxidants in the form of cocoa chews. The healthy skin chocolate soft chews are manufactured by Genuine Health. Three of these chews provide 329 milligrams of cocoa antioxidants with approximately three times less calories, two times less sugar, and six times less fat than an equivalent 40-gram serving of dark chocolate. In addition, the healthy skin chocolate soft chews contain 500 milligrams of fish collagen, which has its own anti-skin-aging research from Japan.

These chews provide a research-based dose of cocoa antioxidants. The same cannot be said for the commercial sale of various "skin healthy" candies and gummy-type products purported to include ingredients that support skin health. The Japanese started the trend in 2002 with the introduction of gummy candies for skin purposes, while North American entrepreneurs caught on later. A closer inspection reveals that more than two hundred of these skin candies would be needed to provide therapeutic levels of zinc and selenium for acne. The 375 grams of sugar in that mini-truckload of gummies would obviously negate the value of selenium or zinc. Our advice: pass on the 250-gummy serving required to get the zinc, selenium, and green tea levels likely to make a difference.

Youthful Skin and the Dietary Acid Load

The acid-base unit of pH refers to the numerical scale called potential of hydrogen, or pH. The scale runs from 1 to 14, with 1 being most acidic and 14 most alkaline, or basic. The pH of our bodily systems is tightly regulated, operating near the middle of the pH scale. In the bloodstream, any deviation away from a near-neutral pH may compromise our very survival.

Dietary foods and beverages can play a large role in the pH systems of the human body. Scientists refer to acid- and alkaline-forming foods, meaning the potential a food or beverage has in tipping the scale toward acidity or alkalinity inside the body. Although determining a food's acidity or alkalinity is somewhat complex, it is essentially dictated by the food's potassium and bicarbonates (alkaline) and protein (acidic) content. Sometimes the foods or beverages we might consider to be "acidic," like citrus fruits or tomatoes, are actually quite alkaline in the body due to their mineral and bicarbonate content.

In North America, we have developed a great fondness for acid-forming foods, particularly animal meats, cheeses, grains, soft drinks, and processed foods. As discussed in chapter 1, we have excluded fruits and vegetables from our plates, and, by doing so, we have given up a rich source of alkaline minerals and bicarbonates. We now have a dietary acid load that is some three times higher than that of the hunter-gatherer diets of traditional, isolated communities. This increased dietary acid load is not without consequence to human health and skin aging.

HISTORY OF DIETARY ACID DERMATOLOGICAL CONSIDERATIONS

The delicate balance between acid and alkaline operating conditions in the human body is something dermatologists were well aware of in the 1930s and 1940s. In 1933, Japanese dermatologist Susumu Tsukada showed that a diet high in acid foods caused higher levels of skin sugar, while alkaline foods prevented sharp rises in skin sugars. After all we have discussed about the sugar-induced skin-aging process, you know only too well that preventing prolonged increases in skin sugar levels is a central tenet to *Your Skin, Younger*. Researchers also discovered in the 1930s that a diet heavy in acidic foods can dehydrate the skin. Two older studies in the 1920s found that as many as 40 percent of those with inflammatory skin conditions had states of mild to moderate acidosis, based on 24-hour urine testing.

Dermatologists knew how easy it was to make the internal body more alkaline—eat fruits and vegetables! The influence of acid-alkaline balance on dry, rough, and scaly skin is highlighted in this quote from an old-school dermatology textbook (*Practical Medicine Series* by Oliver Ormsby [1920]): "In nearly all cases, active inflammatory processes cease and the eruption rapidly clears when the urine is rendered alkaline." In other words, change the diet to a more alkaline intake, and the urine becomes more alkaline, along with an improvement in the skin condition.

Another dermatology textbook (*Skin Diseases: Nutrition and Metabolism* by Erich Urbach [1946]) reported an incredible study that showed ultraviolet-induced skin damage and redness is significantly higher on an acid diet than on an alkaline one! Here we have yet another example of groundbreaking work that was almost discarded in the dustbin of history when the profession turned to pharmaceuticals and relegated nutrition to a non-issue. Once again, dermatology was first on the block with an exciting edge in nutritional medicine, an area that is finally getting its just attention.

> Dietary acids from meats, processed grains, and dairy, left unchecked by the absence of alkaline fruits and vegetables, may negatively influence skin sugar levels and susceptibility to UV damage, and can cause cortisol-induced collagen destruction and overall dehydration of the skin.

WHAT YOU CAN DO

Dietary acid load has once again become a buzzword. For example, a diet high in acidic foods and beverages—particularly in the absence of fruits and vegetables—is associated with increased osteoporosis and fracture risk. Since blood pH must be kept near neutral for our very survival, calcium and magnesium are removed from the bone to buffer, or neutralize, a continuously acidic dietary influence. That calcium and magnesium are subsequently lost in urine. Once acidic meals high in meats, dairy, and processed grain become the rule rather than the exception, an appreciable loss of minerals from the bone matrix will occur.

Furthermore, cells that make bone slow down normal activity in acidic environments. Even a modest change to a more alkaline diet has been shown to be associated with a 50 percent reduction in fracture risk. As mentioned earlier, healthy and fully mineralized bones are an essential component to youthful skin, because bone loss contributes to the visible signs of aging, particularly facial sagging.

An acidic diet is also linked to increased body weight, increased waist circumference, and various markers of cardiovascular disease, including elevated cholesterol and hypertension. An individual whose urine is more alkaline is more likely to have a greater percentage of lean body mass.

ACID DIET AND ACID RAIN ON YOUR COLLAGEN

Obviously, it would be very tempting to ascribe health-promoting associations with alkaline fruits and vegetables to the fact that such diets are subsequently greater in antioxidants and fiber, and contain fewer calories overall. No doubt this is true. However, consider that in 2003, Swiss researchers discovered an important physiological change induced by an acidic, fast-food-type diet—a change that has enormous implications for the health of your collagen. They found that nine days of an acidic diet significantly elevated the stress hormone cortisol. When the researchers neutralized the Western diet with bicarbonate supplements, the cortisol levels dropped down to normal.

Since cortisol is the acid rain that eats away at your collagen, it might be helpful to think of an alkaline diet as a very powerful umbrella. Remember that chronically elevated cortisol contributes to the cycle of inflammation and oxidative stress, and it also disturbs immune function and mood states. Obviously the cortisol connection makes pH an important consideration for the current and future state of your skin.

The lesson here may be less about the acid foods themselves and more about the importance of neutralization with fruits and vegetables or dehydrated colorful plant-based supplements. In other words, the absence of alkaline fruits and vegetables is what really gets us into trouble with our current dietary acid load.

We began this section by making note of the ability of super-foods supplements to contribute to alkaline intake and put a dent in the overall acid load. It really seems like common sense: since the better super-foods are essentially plant-based whole foods with fruits, vegetables, and herbs, wouldn't they have an alkaline influence in the body? They do. A recent study showed that a super-food supplement with dehydrated plant foods significantly changed the pH of first-morning urine. With no other dietary changes, the food supplement made the urine more alkaline after fourteen days of use.

First-morning urine pH has been established as a reliable surrogate marker for the state of acid-alkaline balance in the human body. In your efforts at maintaining youthful skin, measuring urinary pH is an inexpensive investment. Research shows that commercially available litmus paper provides an accurate assessment of pH, equal to that of the dipsticks doctors use. Since a number of health consequences are linked to an overly acidic diet, not the least of which are crumbling dermal structures, testing your pH and supplementing with a quality super-food formula may be worthwhile.

> Super-food powders rich in a variety of dehydrated, plant-based ingredients can provide an internal alkaline balance and help to negate the dehydration and dermal destruction induced by our typical top-heavy acidic diet.

Energizing Your Skin Cells

The functioning of a human skin cell, and ultimately the structure of the skin, is only as good as its energy supply. Cells require a steady supply of nutrients to fuel up for the many jobs that they do—defensive work, repair jobs, regeneration of new cells, and, on the larger scale, actually breathing life into us. As we discussed in chapter 1, human skin cells are constantly doing heavy lifting and backbreaking work in our defense. If there were a medal of honor for a human cell, it would surely go to skin cells.

To function on the front lines of defense, skin cells require massive amounts of energy. The cellular unit responsible for energy production is called the mitochondria. Each of our mitochondrion is like a fully rechargeable AAA battery that uses nutritional components to operate in high gear. When we are young, the mitochondria is very efficient and can run on poor nutritional quality. However, through the aging process, its efficiency declines, and mitochondria becomes less forgiving of our poor selection of dietary choices. Fast food and other nutrient-deficient foods provide only low-grade raw materials for energy production.

When the skin-aging process starts in earnest in mid-life and beyond, the demand for energy production for defense, repair, and regeneration reaches an all-time high. To make matters worse, when the mitochondrial function starts to decline, it actually increases the formation of free radicals and contributes to the oxidative stress burden in the skin.

> Here's the bottom line: a diminished supply of skin energy is highly associated with the visible signs of aging.

Skin-care companies are working hard to develop topical formulations that help to support the functioning of mitochondria. There are also hints that the oral administration of mitochondrial-supporting nutrients can help curb the skin-aging process.

Yutaka Ashida, PhD, and colleagues reported in 2004 that the oral administration of 60 milligrams of Co-enzyme Q_{10} (CoQ_{10}) daily for three months reduced the volume and depth of eye wrinkles. The supplement also increased the total surface area around the eyes that was free from wrinkles. The same group then did experimental studies to see if the oral CoQ_{10} actually reached the skin. Sure enough, the oral administration of CoQ_{10} increased epidermal levels by an astounding 194 percent. Interestingly, most other organs did not see a significant increase in CoQ_{10} levels, indicating that it makes a beeline for its frontline work in the skin. In addition to its role as a strong antioxidant in the skin, CoQ_{10} plays a critical role in the production of mitochondrial energy.

The CoQ_{10} study provides evidence that other nutrients that help maximize mitochondrial function may also have a place in beauty from the inside out. Since many of the B vitamins are essential for the production of energy within the battery, maybe those old advertisements promoting B vitamins for a youthful skin weren't so wrong after all.

Inadequate intake of zinc, one of the most important skin nutrients, has been shown to contribute to mitochondrial decline. An estimated half of the adult population may be deficient in at least one nutrient that otherwise supports mitochondrial function.

Omega-3 fatty acids are also important in mitochondrial functioning. Other specific dietary supplements known to improve energy production in human cells are: α-lipoic acid, acetyl-L-carnitine, creatine, taurine, ribose, quercetin, rhodiola, grape extracts (with the natural chemical resveratrol), and ginkgo biloba. Note that the common thread among most of these ingredients is that they act as strong antioxidants.

Supplementation with a mitochondria cocktail including these ingredients may be of value in keeping your cells energized and highly functioning. In keeping with our theme that a wrinkle is not just a wrinkle, but a reflection of inner health, consider that mitochondrial cocktails of these supplements (especially CoQ_{10}, α-lipoic acid, and acetyl-L-carnitine) have been shown to be helpful in a number of age-related diseases, including neurodegenerative diseases.

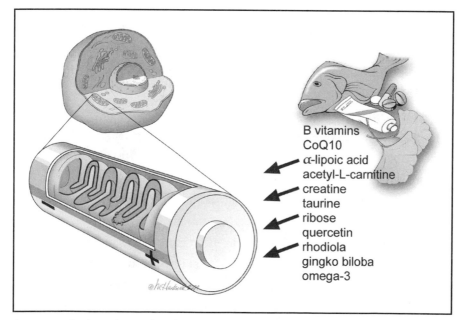

B vitamins
CoQ10
α-lipoic acid
acetyl-L-carnitine
creatine
taurine
ribose
quercetin
rhodiola
gingko biloba
omega-3

As we age, the loss of energy in the mitochondria of the skin can contribute to the visible signs of aging. Nutritional support for the skin's batteries is essential in the limitation of the skin's aging process.

Remember that this is more than a superficial issue; mitochondrial decay is at the core of most diseases of aging. Not surprisingly, a number of these mitochondria-supporting chemicals and herbs can now be found in the ingredient list of the natural topical preparations we will discuss in the next chapter. Finally, exercise is known to be one of the best ways to preserve the structure and function of the mitochondria through the aging process.

Ceramides

If you have a good memory, you will recall from chapter 1 that the stratum corneum is a wafer-thin layer within the epidermis, a brick-and-mortar structure enlisted with the incredible responsibility of providing a barrier and maintaining skin hydration. The healthy moisture in glowing, well-hydrated skin is a reflection of a well-preserved brick wall. The mortar within the brick wall is essentially a lipid, or fat, substance made up in large part by a special class of lipids called ceramides.

For the past two decades, high-end topical cosmetic formulations have included ceramides for good reason. Levels of ceramides decline with age as well as during the winter months, and low levels of skin ceramides are, in turn, associated with dry and inflamed skin. A reduction in skin ceramide levels is highly associated with the development of visible signs of aging through the aging process. UV exposure also releases ceramides from their home in the mortar of the stratum-corneum wall.

To make matters worse, ceramides are not benign fatty substances. They are very active, which was discovered only recently. When levels of ceramides start to drop, they send out signals to turn up the dial on inflammatory chemicals—obviously the last thing you need when trying to maintain youthful skin. Apparently, a drop in skin ceramides is interpreted as danger, and one way the body responds to danger is by turning on inflammatory pathways. However, in the case of low ceramide levels, inflammatory chemicals only serve to further disturb the skin barrier.

The good news is that not only are topical ceramide-containing formulas available, but new research also shows that orally consumed ceramides can make a big difference in the integrity of the skin barrier. Ceramides occur naturally in a number of plants, most notably the oils of rice bran and wheat germ. New technology has allowed concentrated ceramides to be derived from these healthy oils.

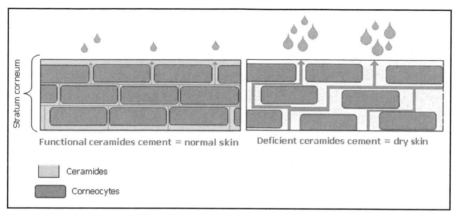

Ceramides are the mortar of the "brick wall" layer within the epidermis. They ensure cohesion of the "bricks," the keratin-rich corneocytes. Natural plant-based ceramides such as LipoWheat help to maintain the great epidermal wall. LipoWheat is a trademark of LaviPharm Group.

At one time, the notion of orally consumed ceramides to promote beauty from the inside out was scoffed at—until Japanese researchers showed in 2007 that orally consumed plant ceramides could improve hydration in the stratum corneum by 253 percent over placebo in human volunteers. The study indicated that oral ceramides can be effective after three weeks of use. In addition, a recent report from the Satou Hospital in Osaka, Japan, suggests that oral administration of plant-derived ceramides can turn down the dial on inflammatory chemicals in young children with chronic skin inflammation. Since oral ceramides can both lower inflammation and keep the skin well hydrated, they are one of the most exciting advances in the maintenance of youthful skin in recent years. Currently the most highly researched plant-based ceramide used in oral formulations is that known as LipoWheat.

Superoxide Dismutase

Recall from our earlier discussions that skin anti-aging pioneer, Manhattan dermatologist Irwin I. Lubowe, MD, advocated for the use of oral superoxide dismutase (SOD) to prevent skin aging. SOD was theorized to work because it is one of our most important antioxidants and one of the greatest protectors of the mitochondria. New experimental genetic studies indicate that high levels of SOD in mitochondria will extend survival in living organisms.

Lubowe's skin-specific advice is also supported by recent studies on a new SOD supplement. Researchers showed that a specially coated SOD, taken orally for one month, increased the amount of UV rays necessary to cause burning in sun-sensitive adult volunteers. The results supported a previous French study that used 500 milligrams of the coated SOD and also found it to be effective in reducing UV-induced skin damage. Since a significant portion of orally administered SOD is broken down in the digestive tract, coating it with a wheat protein increases absorption by 57 percent. Currently the most highly absorbed form of oral SOD is commercially available as Super Glisodin.

One way to maintain healthy SOD levels in addition to specific supplementation is to take a super-food supplement. The natural antioxidants in colorful foods will lower the demand for SOD and keep levels high in the skin.

Silicon

The mineral silicon, not to be confused with synthetic silicone, is found in many structures of the human body, most notably bones, hair, skin, and nails. Silicon is a mineral that hasn't had much respect in the annals of nutritional medicine. We know how important calcium, magnesium, and zinc are, yet silicon is often bypassed as having little consequence to human health. In reality, a dietary deficiency of silicon can decrease the manufacture of both collagen and the GAGs that support collagen structures. Silicon seems to hold the GAGs together, like a joint or brace to the long pieces of scaffolding.

Major food sources of silicon include whole grains, especially those with the bran portion intact. High-bran breakfast cereal and brown rice are particularly rich in silicon, although other plant-based foods such as raisins, bananas, carrots, and green beans are also very high in silicon. Once again, it's the same old chestnut: whole grains and deeply colored plant foods are the skin's best friend. Since silicon stimulates the collagen in bone, a diet high in silicon is associated with greater bone-mineral density in adults.

SILICON AND THE ASIAN DIET

The silicon rich, plant-food diet of Asian nations is purported to be one of the reasons why the rates of osteoporosis and hip fractures are lower in many Asian countries. Knowing that dietary silica is absorbed and converted into an active form of silicon, one could also make an argument for silicon as one of the many reasons for a lower rate of the visible signs of aging in older Asian adults. The average silicon intake among Japanese adults is about 40 percent higher than that of North Americans.

Silicon exists in food (and some herbs such as horsetail extract) as silica. For years, silica was assumed to have very poor absorption from the gastrointestinal tract. But that urban legend is not true. Dietary silica is absorbed and converted into the active form of silicon, called orthosilicic acid (OA). You want that active form of silicon for gorgeously firm, glowing skin. The average dietary intake of silicon is about 28 milligrams among North Americans. A little less than half of that is actually absorbed and converted into the important OA form of silicon.

Recently, a stable form of active silicon has become available, and it has been shown to be very well absorbed. The OA form of silicon is stabilized with choline, and experimental studies showed that supplementation with this unique formula can increase collagen formation in the skin of animals. In a clinical study published in the *Archives of Dermatological Research* (2005), researchers from Belgium showed that 10 milligrams of oral OA (consumed for twenty weeks) significantly decreased skin roughness and improved elasticity of the skin versus placebo. These are impressive results, considering that an additional 10 milligrams of silicon is not much, although it does bring consumers up into the range of the typical Asian diet.

What to Take?

In the sea of some thirty thousand different supplements in North America, confusion and outlandish claims abound. Walking into a health-food store, you may feel like you need a PhD in nutritional sciences to cut through the hype and find supplements helpful in promoting youthful skin. We have covered a fair bit of ground in this chapter regarding specific supplements with the potential to promote youthful skin and keep the visible signs of aging in check. So-called skingestibles can make a difference. Now it's time to put this research into perspective and create a priority placement of the supplements that can feed the skin. As new research on oral skin supplements and topical nutrients emerges, it will be added to author Alan Logan's website at http://www.drlogan.com. A cautionary reminder: skin food in the form of supplements is not a substitute for making every effort to enrich the diet with a wide variety of colorful fruits, vegetables, whole grains, culinary herbs, fermented foods such as yogurt, and fish and seafood. The word supplement should be taken literally—it is an add-on to the best of dietary intentions. It is not called a dietary *substitute*, but rather a dietary *supplement*—and supplements will never substitute for a healthy diet. That said, let's consider our supplement plan for youthful skin.

QUALITY MULTIVITAMIN-MINERAL FORMULA

This is the cornerstone of any supplement plan. We are not alone in recommending a daily multivitamin. Harvard's School of Public Health states clearly on its website in 2009 that "a daily multivitamin is a great nutrition insurance policy." They urge consumers not to be put off by all the conflicting studies on vitamins that can "make your head swirl." Multi formulas are not going to prevent cancer, colds, viral infections, heart attacks, mental health disorders, or even facial wrinkles.

A multivitamin represents an inexpensive way to cover some of the voids that may exist in a substellar diet.

Based on the realities of North American dietary habits as described in chapter 1, we maintain that a multivitamin-mineral formula should be first on the list. Choose one without unnecessary food dyes, such as FD&C yellow #6 aluminum lake, and other additives. Avoid mega-doses of vitamins and minerals beyond the upper limits set by the U.S. Institute of Medicine and Health Canada. Consider that some daily multi preparations now contain additional, so-called added-value ingredients for the maintenance of youthful skin, including fish collagen and lycopene, as discussed above. Our philosophy is to keep it simple and trim down the need to take bags full of supplements—so if a multivitamin contains extras like fish collagen and lycopene, that's great.

FISH OIL WITH EPA

The current combined daily intake of the skin-friendly omega-3 fatty acids EPA and DHA is around 130 milligrams. For most North Americans, that is not even close to where we need to be. The international panel of lipid experts has recommended a minimum of 650 milligrams of combined EPA and DHA daily. If you do not consume salmon, sardines, mackerel, and anchovies regularly, and you want youthful skin, supplementation is highly recommended. As previously discussed, EPA is the anti-inflammatory component of omega-3. It does the lion's share of work in protecting collagen. For optimal protection against the skin-aging process, consider taking at least 1,000 milligrams of EPA daily. For additional collagen protection and to improve elasticity of the skin, consider adding 250 to 500 milligrams of gamma-linolenic acid (GLA) from borage or evening primrose oil. Some studies show that taking EPA along with GLA may provide enhanced results.

SKIN ANTI-AGING NUTRIENT HIGHLIGHT: EICOSAPENTAENOIC ACID

What is it?
Eicosapentaenoic acid (EPA) is an important omega-3 fatty acid found in fish and seafood—particularly oily ocean fish such as sardines, mackerel, and anchovies.

Why is it of value?
EPA is arguably the greatest anti-inflammatory found in nature. It dampens the production of the major collagen-destroying

chemical, PGE2. EPA also lowers inflammatory cytokines, which are implicated in the skin-aging process. Taken orally, EPA has been shown to improve skin-barrier function and improve elasticity. Topically and orally, EPA can reduce UV-induced skin cell damage. Topical EPA from deodorized fish oil has now become commercially available from Genuine Health. The final clinical trial results are pending; however, preliminary investigations indicate that over 70 percent of women using the topical products containing EPA report improvements in satisfaction with skin. Firmness, texture, tone, and hydration improved, while fine lines, wrinkles, dark circles, puffiness decreased. The improvements were not minor; there was an average 43 percent improvement in overall ratings of skin satisfaction. In addition, human studies show that between 1 and 2 grams of oral EPA has a mood-regulating effect that may assist with resilience to stress.

MARINE FISH COLLAGEN

Since healthy collagen structure is at the heart of skin-aging, we have included marine collagen in our top priority list. Shoot for 500 to 1,000 milligrams of marine collagen in a supplement. Research supports the use of fish collagen in humans, and it appears to be one of the most important ways to provide the building blocks for healthy skin collagen. Powdered collagen supplements are available as stand-alone supplements, and fish collagen also can be found in multivitamin and multi-ingredient skingestibles.

Check labels and bypass products that only offer a smidgen of fish collagen. As mentioned, Genuine Health (http://www.genuinehealth.com) offers healthy skin chocolate soft chews that contain the high-antioxidant cocoa extract shown to improve blood flow to the skin, hydration of the skin, and increased dermal thickness. Eat three of the chews, and you'll also get 500 milligrams of fish collagen from cod and 6 milligrams of lycopene. Sweetened primarily with brown rice syrup, each chew only has about 2 grams of sugar and 30 calories.

QUALITY PROBIOTIC

Having devoted an entire chapter to gut health for the maintenance of youthful skin, it shouldn't be shocking that we place probiotics on our priority list. Probiotics can lower inflammation and oxidative stress throughout the body, which is why you should take a probiotic for healthy skin. As mentioned, the challenge is deciding which probiotic to take and how much you need. Among our top choices are *Bifidobacterium* infantis 35624 (commercially available as Align from Procter & Gamble) and *Lactobacillus* plantarum 299V (LactoFlamX from Metagenics) because these strains can lower inflammation and oxidative stress in the far reaches of the body when orally consumed.

Further information on yogurts, supplements, and how to obtain these and other strains with great potential in protecting the skin can be found in the Appendices. Probiotic yogurts are also listed. Note that most experts suggest that at least 1 billion colony-forming units are required as an effective dose for a probiotic.

PROBIOTIC PICKS

Yogurt and Yogurt Drinks:
- Activia (Dannon Company)
- DanActive (Dannon Company)
- Rachel's Vitality (Pomegranate/Acai) and Exotic (Pomegranate/ Blueberry)
- Stonyfield Farm Organic
- Yakult (Yakult Honsha Company)

Supplements:
- Align (Procter & Gamble)—*Bifidobacterium* infantis 35624
- Bifido Factor (Natren)—*Bifidobacterium* bifidum Mayloth
- Culturelle (Amerifit Brands)—*Lactobacillus* GG
- LactoFlamX (Metagenics)—*Lactobacillus* plantarum 299V
- Probifia (Nature's Way)—*Bifidobacterium* longum BB536

Note: With commercial yogurt and yogurt drinks, be cautious about overconsuming the added sugars. Low-fat plain yogurts typically contain only 15 to 18 grams of natural sugars found in dairy. Some yogurts on the market contain more than 40 grams of total sugar, so watch out for those.

SUPER-FOOD

Why take a bag full of individual skin-friendly supplements like green tea, lycopene, red wine antioxidants, ginger, turmeric, lutein, blood orange, and zeaxanthin when a powdered whole-food formula will cover the antioxidant bases in one simple and convenient place? We consider a high-quality super-food formula to be akin to a daily multivitamin, except that the nutritional void being filled is that of plant-based antioxidants, the so-called phytochemicals.

To be clear, our recommended version of a super-food is one that contains a wide variety of colorful fruits, vegetables, or whole grains, or a combination of these, in powder form. Sometimes the word super-food is used to signify a single food, such as acai or blueberries, yet we refer to products that include these and many other high antioxidant foods as well. As mentioned, our philosophy when it comes to supplements is one of simplicity. We ask ourselves, how can we pare down to the basics? Taking a super-food powder negates the need to take multiple antioxidant pills, and the synergy of the whole plant foods with water removed is second only to healthy foods served up on a plate.

With the ability of super-food powders to alkalinize the body, they represent one of the most efficient ways to keep cortisol in check and stop the onslaught of acid rain on the collagen. The antioxidants and herbal extracts that often appear in super-food formulas are very important for the maintenance of healthy mitochondria in your skin cells. Some super-food formulas are skin specific and include a number of the mitochondria cocktail nutrients and other ingredients discussed above. Fish collagen; rice bran or wheat germ ceramides; tomato extract with lycopene; cocoa flavanols; and silica from horsetail extract are all examples that show up in some super-food formulas as added-value ingredients.

TOLERABLE UPPER LIMITS OF ADULT DIETARY REFERENCE INTAKES

One cautionary note: when taking multiple supplements, including multivitamins and other skin supplements with added vitamins and minerals, be cautious regarding the tolerable upper limits of total daily vitamins and minerals. Sometimes more is not necessarily better, and that is certainly the case with three skin-friendly minerals—zinc, selenium, and chromium. At or below the tolerable upper limits, these minerals are the skin's best friend; above those limits, they can compromise the immune system and cause internal toxicities.

Folic acid	1,000 mcg
Niacin	35 mg
Vitamin B$_6$	100 mg
Vitamin A	3,000 mcg
Vitamin C	2,000 mg
Vitamin D	50 mcg
Vitamin E	1,000 mg
Choline	3,500 mg
Boron	20 mg
Calcium	2,500 mg
Copper	10 mg
Fluoride	10 mg
Iodine	1,100 mcg
Iron	45 mg
Magnesium	350 mg
Manganese	11 mg
Molybdenum	2,000 mcg
Nickel	1 mg

Phosphorus	4,000 mg
Selenium	400 mcg
Vanadium	1.8 mg
Zinc	40 mg
Water	3.7 L male; 2.7 L female

Source: National Academy of Sciences, Institute of Medicine

Our basic supplementation plan is actually quite simple. Of course, you can take any of a number of different supplements for skin health. Indeed, the sky is the limit when it comes to choices. By keeping your list to a simple five supplements, you'll have a much greater chance of compliance. All of your authors know from clinical experience that, with each addition to a routine—whether it is prescription drugs, topicals, or supplements, or some combination of these—the rate of compliance will go down.

In short, the more supplements you set out to take for skin, the less likely you will be to do so over the long term. Our top five choices for younger skin from the inside out are chosen based on their ability to preserve collagen, protect against UV damage, reduce inflammation, and improve hydration of the skin. For more details, see the Appendices.

7

Skin Food II:
Natural Topicals

Topical preparations for medicinal and cosmetic purposes have been used since time immemorial. Many of the ingredients used as beautifying agents over the years were formulated from foods and herbs. As mentioned in chapter 4, Romans and ancient Egyptians used milk-based facial washes, likely to take advantage of the naturally occurring acids within milk. Others used fermented milk products topically, including a bubbly "milk champagne" probiotic liquid that resembles modern kefir.

Fundamentally, our contemporary cosmetics are quite similar to many of the formulations used by the ancient Romans. Indeed, when a very rare, unopened Roman cosmetic was excavated and evaluated by scientists in 2004, they were quite surprised with the similarities in the natural chemical ingredients as compared to modern moisturizing creams. The Romans used olive oil, botanical extracts, culinary herbs, berries, almonds, beeswax, and other plant-based ingredients with a great degree of sophistication.

By the early twentieth century, most scientists considered these natural concoctions to have little value for anything other than the temporary maintenance of moisture and other superficial influences. Experts scoffed at the notion that the deeper layers of the skin could be "fed" by topical nutrients for beauty because the skin was viewed as a one-way street of expulsion. Sweat, sebum, sloughing of cells, and secretion of waste are all outward bound.

History of Topical Skin Products

With only a few exceptions, the skin was considered impermeable to food-based material until Karl Stejskal, MD, of Vienna showed otherwise in 1926. He first showed that olive oil can penetrate the skin and make it into the body. Over the next few years, he experimented with a variety of different carbohydrates, proteins, and fats, showing unexpected skin penetration for even some of the larger, food-based molecules.

Eventually his work made headlines in North America (*Popular Science* April, 1929, read: "Physician feeds patient through pores in skin"), and he endorsed a line of topical "Skin Food" from the Tokalon Company. Stejskal was reported to have studied the topical Skin Food in older women in a hospital setting in Vienna. He claimed it promoted more youthful skin after six weeks. This first-generation topical Skin Food included proteins and polysaccharides derived from the dermal layer of animal skin.

Still, most dermatologists did not see any credibility in so-called skin foods (food-based nutrients applied topically), and they were mostly dismissed as a fad. Although some forms of skin food, including royal jelly and seaweed, would explode onto the topical skin-care market in the 1950s, scientists would dismiss these, too, as fads with no credibility. Referring to royal jelly (the food delivered to the queen bee by its worker bees and highly touted for its skin-rejuvenating properties), one industry chemist stated in *Time* magazine (June 16, 1958): "It is a fad and does nothing for the skin."

Science would prove him wrong and, as we will discuss, new studies do show the value of topical royal jelly and seaweed extracts. Nevertheless, it would take decades before scientists would apply good science to topical nutrition for youthful skin. Indeed it wasn't until 1976 that researchers proved that the topical application of essential fatty acids (EFA) can overcome a dietary EFA deficiency in hospitalized patients using IV feeding—proving that Stejskal was right in his suggestion that dietary components can be absorbed.

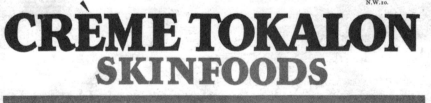

Younger Every Morning!

Try this recipe tonight

Thanks to this marvellous discovery, wrinkles can be made to disappear and the skin regain its youthful beauty.

Science has long known that it is the loss of certain vital elements from the skin which causes wrinkles and faded skin. These precious substances can now be restored by the amazing, recently found method of Dr. Stejskal of the University of Vienna.

Extracted from the skin of carefully selected young animals by Prof. Dr. Stejskal, 'Biocel,' the active principle of living cells, is contained in Tokalon Rose Skinfood. By its use an aged, faded skin can quickly be nourished and rejuvenated—sallow complexion made clear and fresh.

Try Tokalon Biocel Skinfood to-night. Even by to-morrow morning you will see an amazing difference in the clearness and freshness of your skin. In the daytime use Tokalon Vanishing Skinfood (non-greasy); whitening tonic and astringent. After one month's use in this way you will look at least ten years younger.

VANISHING SKINFOOD (White). Tubes 6d. Jars 1/-.
BIOCEL SKINFOOD (Rose) Tubes 6d. Jars 1/3.

FREE: By arrangement with the manufacturers any reader of this paper may now obtain a de Luxe Beauty Outfit containing the new Tokalon Skinfood Creams (Rose for the evening; White for the day). It contains also trial packets of Tokalon 'Mousse of Cream' Powder. Send 3d. in stamps to cover cost of postage, packing and other expenses. Address: Tokalon, Ltd., **(Dept. 431L),** Chase Road, London, N.W.10.

CRÈME TOKALON SKINFOODS

Karl Stejskal's Skin Food was the most popular physician-endorsed cosmetic in Europe in the 1920s and 1930s.

Looking at it from a modern vantage, Stejskal's use of olive oil and other unsaturated fats was almost certainly the secret to his success with topical skin foods. As we will discuss, only recently have researchers discovered that certain fats, particularly polyunsaturated fats and fish oil, help to improve the penetration of other drugs and nutrients through the skin.

Niche Market No More

While natural cosmetics certainly received no embrace from mainstream dermatology, and scientific investigations lagged far behind marketing claims, the counterculture movement of the late 1960s and early 1970s fueled a small but growing niche. Small independent manufacturers paved the way with plant-based organic cosmetics, many of which included ingredients now known to positively influence the condition of human skin through the aging process. *Time* magazine published a feature article on the growing popularity of natural cosmetics with fruit and berry extracts, sesame, and wheat germ oils (January 18, 1971), and from that point on, there was no turning back.

What started as a small, fringe movement with a few pioneers would ultimately explode into the massive $7 billion-plus global natural and organic cosmetics market we have today. Along the way from its humble origins in the tiny health-food stores of the 1970s, the market would see some of the biggest cosmetic corporations jumping onto the natural skin-food bandwagon. When the corporate conglomerates jumped on, the aforementioned bandwagon was filled to the brim with previously skeptical scientists, researchers, and consulting dermatologists. Incredibly, some dermatologists went from vocal opposition to the idea of skin foods to becoming corporate cosmetic spokespersons for natural ingredients within the span of a decade.

What changed in the interim was the science behind the plant-based cosmetic movement. Corporations jumped on the bandwagon with sack loads of cash—money that would propel research and proper scientific inquiry into the use of topical skin foods. Not surprisingly, research would show that nutrient and herbal-based ingredients that have anti-inflammatory, antioxidant, and anti-glycating properties would be of value to aging skin. Topical ingredients that support and defend the dermal structures (such as collagen and GAGs) would also be shown to be among the top picks, as well as nutrients and herbs that support the mitochondria. Of course, our favorite essential fatty acids, the omega-3 from fish and GLA from borage oil, as well as lipid-based ceramides would also get the proverbial gold star for protection against aging skin.

Vitamin A

Topical vitamin A within cold cream was launched in the late 1930s as a Skin-Vitamin formula to improve dry, rough skin and to maintain a youthful appearance. Vitamin A can indeed improve skin appearance. In addition to having anti-acne properties, specific forms of the vitamin can also produce smoother, less wrinkled skin with continued use. Retinol is a naturally occurring vitamin A that is fat soluble and capable of penetrating the dermis. Once inside the skin, it can be converted into the biologically active form of vitamin A, called retinoic acid.

The retinoids that make up the vitamin A family are a dream for the skin. They have antioxidant activity and turn on the production of collagen and GAGs, and very importantly, they turn down the dial on MMPs (enzymes that destroy collagen). Clearly, retinoids are the skin's best friend, and they sit at the core of any topical anti-aging formula. The more potent retinoic acid is available from your dermatologist by prescription, although retinol is also available in over the counter preparations. Studies have confirmed that non-prescription topical retinol can provide significant benefit in reducing wrinkles and increasing dermal GAGs.

Vitamins C and E

Both of these important vitamins confer antioxidant protection on collagen when topically applied. While both vitamins have individual research to support their inclusion in natural topical skin formulas, they are, with good reason, rarely applied alone. The combination of the two is the most common form of delivery because they work in synergy. Vitamin C can preserve vitamin E levels, while vitamin E helps to preserve all antioxidant stores in the skin. To highlight the synergy of the two vitamins, consider a study published in the *Journal of the American Academy of Dermatology* (2003) that showed that the combo was twice as valuable to the skin in UV protection as either of the antioxidant vitamins was alone.

The inclusion of other plant-based antioxidants—such as ferulic acid from rice bran or wheat extracts in topical formulas—can also increase the antioxidant potential of these vitamins. Either alone or together, the topical application of vitamins C and E improves the appearance of aged skin, protects against UV damage, and, based on instrumentation studies, improves the texture and collagen structures within the skin. Note that vitamins C and E are normally provided in the more stable ester forms for skin application.

Keep in mind that the topical use of these particular vitamins is not a quick fix. It can take months of use to see marked improvements. Relying on vitamins A, C, and E in topical form as the sole measure to maintain youthful skin is likely to be met with disappointment overall. Sure, there are encouraging studies, but combining these vitamins with the other food-based antioxidant and anti-inflammatory ingredients discussed below will be far more likely to provide a meaningful difference.

B Vitamins

Despite a long history of use as a beauty vitamin from within, and despite the knowledge that some B vitamins support collagen formation, the external application of B vitamins is a surprisingly recent phenomenon. Researchers began tinkering with topical B vitamins in the 1960s and showed that some of the vitamin family members have anti-inflammatory properties in the skin. However, scientists generally considered that the strict water-soluble nature and large size of these vitamins negated their ability to have any significant impact on skin health.

In recent years, dermatological scientists have turned this thinking on its head. Many of the B vitamins do permeate through the skin, and some can even make it into the bloodstream in significant amounts. Well-designed human studies have shown that topical vitamin B_{12} is highly effective in reducing skin inflammation when applied as a cream, and other human studies have highlighted the anti-aging properties of two other topically applied B vitamins—vitamin B_3 and folic acid.

The topical application of vitamin B_3 (as nicotinic acid or niacinamide) can prevent water loss from the skin. It can also stimulate the production of ceramides and the keratin in the epidermis. Vitamin B$_3$ is like an epidermal bricklayer because it has a positive influence on both the bricks and the mortar. In addition, it has been shown to have anti-inflammatory properties when topically applied. Not only that, but topical vitamin B$_3$ reduces the appearance of fine lines and wrinkles (including eye wrinkles!) and can produce a more uniform color to the skin. The latter attribute should not be underestimated as some studies indicate that a non-uniform skin tone with blotches and hyperpigmentation is perceived as a major contributor to a more aged skin appearance, right up there with wrinkles.

An added value of vitamin B$_3$ is that it can help prevent the usual suppression of the immune system after UV exposure when taken either orally or topically. Note that in the beauty realm, the form of B$_3$ used is typically niacinomide. Dosing with oral B$_3$ as the niacin form found in some vitamin supplements may lead to an uncomfortable flushing reaction in the skin.

When inflammation is ongoing in the skin (and with our dietary habits and stressors these days, when is it not?), the skin steps up its demand for the B vitamin folic acid. We know that after UV exposure, the skin's demand for folic acid increases, likely because one of folate's most important roles is in the protection and repair of the DNA in our cells and in the formation of new cells.

In a study published in the *Journal of Cosmetic Dermatology* (2008), German researchers showed that topical folic acid (along with creatine, which we will discuss later) protected human skin against UV damage, reduced the volume of wrinkles, and increased skin firmness relative to the control. Based on the grading system, there was a significant decrease in fine lines and wrinkles around the eyes, and the skin was smoother after eight weeks of use. While the role of creatine, a nutrient which supports the energy production in skin cells cannot be dismissed, it is almost certain that more studies on topical folic acid will roll out soon. Topical B vitamins are undoubtedly here to stay as part of topical skin foods.

Essential Fats

We have placed great emphasis on the ability of certain fats to turn down the dial on inflammation and promote youthful, glowing, and well-hydrated skin. Thankfully, new technology has emerged to deodorize fish oil, leaving the important omega-3 fatty acids safely intact while allowing you not to smell like an unattended fish tank. Along with technological advances in the processing of fish oil has come a new wave of research on topical fish oils. The key omega-3 fatty acid EPA, in particular, has emerged as the skin's best fatty-acid friend.

Recall that EPA is the most important anti-inflammatory omega-3 fatty acid from fish and seafood. Topical EPA reduces inflammatory skin conditions such as psoriasis. It also reduces UV damage, lowering the MMPs that usually destroy collagen and preventing the thickening and crusting of the outer layer of skin (the epidermis) that usually occurs after UV exposure. An additional benefit derived from topical EPA is its ability to prevent the usual suppression of the immune system that occurs as a result of UV exposure.

The exciting results of topical EPA cannot be extrapolated to other plant forms of omega-3 fatty acids. Japanese researchers from Nagoya City University showed that, in topical form, plant-based omega-3 (alpha-linolenic acid) does not protect against UV damage. The dietary form was effective at protecting from the inside out, just not the topical. The take-home message from the research—that fish oil-based EPA is the UV-protecting omega-3—is at odds with the marketing materials of companies that promote topical "omega-3" creams, lotions, and gels for skin.

Many of these companies use cheap alpha-linolenic acid as the omega-3 source without informing consumers that it is not the same as the omega-3 EPA from fish oil. It will not perform in the same way when topically applied. Cutting-edge formulas with fish-derived, deodorized EPA cost more money to manufacture. However, they deliver a direct anti-inflammatory influence to the skin layers. Reputable companies, like Genuine Health, who use deodorized EPA-rich fish oil for skin care will do so from sustainable sources, such as small sardines and anchovies.

Topical application of EPA is clearly effective because the fatty acid has no difficulty moving through the skin layers to do its job. In fact, EPA, fish oil itself, and other healthy fats can actually help other nutrients and drugs to move through the skin layers.

Added value: New EPA omega-3 topical formulas for youthful skin help carry other skin-food nutrients down through the skin layers.

The so-called pull-and-drag effect of EPA and fish oil has been documented a number of times with a variety of different chemicals that would normally have poor permeability through the skin layers due to size. EPA's anti-inflammatory, collagen-protecting, and UV-defending properties—and EPA's ability to carry other antioxidants and nutrients through the skin—make it and deodorized fish oil the most important and exciting advances in topical anti-aging skin care since the discovery of retinoids.

In the excitement surrounding the application of topical EPA for the maintenance of youthful skin, we cannot overlook the importance of GLA from primrose or borage oils. GLA also has anti-inflammatory activity and can help push production of the ceramides that help build up the epidermal barrier. Topical GLA from either GLA or borage oil can improve the epidermal barrier function and diminish the dehydration common to aging skin.

In what has to be one of the most unique studies we have reviewed for this entire book, researchers from Japan reported in the *Journal of Dermatology* (2007) that wearing undershirts specially coated with borage oil (versus shirts with no borage oil) for two weeks reduced inflammation and improved skin hydration in those with inflammatory dermatitis. Incredibly, the borage oil was chemically bonded to the organic cotton undershirts and designed for gradual release into the inflamed skin. That is surely the most unique delivery format of GLA to date!

Other Fatty Friends

Three other members of the lipid family have been making waves in the topical anti-aging skin-care world: ceramides, squalene, and phosphatidylserine (PS).

CERAMIDES

We have addressed the oral use of ceramides, and the results with topical application are no less impressive. Remember that the ceramides are the mortar in the great wall of the epidermis. They keep the water inside skin, and we inevitably lose this mortar through the aging process. Youthful skin is well hydrated because of ceramides, but as we lose the ceramides through aging, our skin becomes dry and dehydrated. UV exposure can release the ceramides from their normal housing in the epidermis. It makes sense to replace the ceramides for the maintenance of youthful skin, and big-name cosmetic companies have been using synthetic ceramides for years.

Thankfully, natural plant-derived ceramides have arrived on the scene, bringing with them other important antioxidants and fats found in the foods of origin. For example, ceramides from wheat germ and rice bran are surrounded by additional antioxidants. Natural plant-based ceramides have recently been shown to keep the skin well hydrated in adult volunteers, increasing hydration by 141 percent over placebo after topical application of rice bran-ceramides.

German researchers reported in 2008 that topical ceramides with vitamins (versus vitamins alone) provide an edge in that they can signal for the manufacture of collagen after UV exposure. The ceramide and vitamin combination also decreased collagen-degrading MMPs after UV exposure in healthy adults. Ceramides, therefore, keep the outer layer of the skin well hydrated and the underlying scaffolding intact in the face of environmental assaults.

SQUALENE

Squalene gets its name from the Latin word for shark (*Squalus*) because it was first isolated in the oils of shark liver. In the early 1950s, researchers discovered that squalene is a key component in the fats that protect the outer surface of the skin. As you can imagine, it didn't take long to get shark liver oil into cosmetics, and some of the more heavily advertised in the late 1950s were selling for $115 a jar—the equivalent of more than $800 today when inflation adjusted! Turns out that squalene is not exclusive to the liver of shark. Appreciable amounts occur in olives and the same skin-friendly oils that provide ceramides—rice bran and wheat germ oils.

There is no doubt about the ability of squalene to act as an emollient, a substance that promotes a soft and smooth feel to the skin. It is rapidly absorbed when applied topically without leaving an oily residue and helps improve hydration. Yet squalene is so much more. It also acts as an important antioxidant, protecting the other fats in the outer layers of skin that may otherwise be susceptible to free-radical damage from the sun, pollution, and electromagnetic radiation. Experimental studies have also shown that topically applied squalene may protect against skin cancer. Thankfully, the days of $800 shark-liver-oil skin creams are over. Natural, plant-based squalene is a relatively inexpensive ingredient in many topical skin foods.

PHOSPHATIDYLSERINE

Phosphatidylserine (PS) is found naturally in soy lecithin and egg yolks, and makes up an important part of the structure of not only skin cells, but all cells. Although best known as a structural component of the walls of skin cells, PS is no wallflower, researchers are starting to learn. Emerging studies suggest that PS acts like an orchestra conductor in its ability to turn on and signal for anti-inflammatory chemicals. It also has direct antioxidant properties.

Still, PS was largely off the radar for cosmetic scientists until Korean researchers published a landmark study in the *Journal of Lipid Research* (2008). They found that topical PS can slow down the activity of the collagen-destroying MMP enzymes after UV exposure in young adults, and it also significantly reduced the production of collagen-damaging inflammatory chemicals. In older skin, the application of topical PS was able to step up collagen formation and decrease the levels of damaging MMPs, regardless of UV exposure.

In other words, PS is not only a topical UV protector; it also steps up collagen formation and slows down collagen destruction through the aging process, even in sun-protected skin. There is no doubt that the combination of essential fatty acids, ceramides, squalene, and PS, collectively used as commercial DermaLipid in topical and oral skin foods, is the fatty family of choice for well-hydrated and young-looking skin.

As mentioned, other skin-friendly dietary fats have been used for centuries to promote healthy appearance and maintain youthful skin. Olive oil in the Mediterranean region and sesame oil in South Asia have long held reputations as oils to enhance beauty when used for facial massage. Sesame and olive oils are both very rich in antioxidants that are now the subject of intense anti-aging research.

A special extract from olives called Olivem 1000 has been shown to act as a barrier against water loss and provide antioxidant and anti-inflammatory support in the skin. One of the major antioxidants found in sesame seeds, sesamol, penetrates into the dermis and protects collagen against UV destruction in experimental studies. Topical olive oil reduces skin cancer and enhances repair mechanisms in the skin due to UV radiation in experimental settings.

Fruit and Dairy Acids

Lactic acid found in fermented dairy products; malic, citric and tartaric acids found in fruits; and glycolic acid found in sugarcane and beets are collectively referred to as alpha-hydroxy acids (AHAs) in cosmetic science. These are weak organic acids, structurally similar to each other regardless of their natural sources. AHAs are found in sour milk and fermented wines. Of course, when ancient Egyptians were using sour milk and upper-class French women of the eighteenth century were using fermented wines for facial rejuvenation, they weren't referring to the process as AHA therapy!

The exact mechanisms of how AHAs work towards skin rejuvenation remain a matter of scientific discussion. But the value of AHAs for the maintenance of healthy, youthful skin is not up for debate. Research has shown a number of ways in which AHAs improve the appearance of aging skin. What is known is that AHAs help to shed the flaky outer layer of the epidermis, which causes wrinkles and fine lines to appear less prominent. AHA use also moisturizes the skin, improves dermal thickness by stimulating collagen production, and significantly improves blood flow to the skin. In addition, AHA therapy can decrease the hyperpigmentation associated with the aging process and improve overall skin tone.

Recently, beta hydroxyl acids (BHAs)—including the salicylic acid found in berries and other plants—have been reported to have similar skin-rejuvenating properties. Caprylic acid derived from coconut is yet another plant-based organic acid that may be helpful in the promotion of youthful skin. Scientists from Europe reported in the *International Journal of Dermatology* (2008) that using AHAs together with retinoids may offer additional skin-rejuvenating support in hydration and elasticity. Keep in mind that the smaller concentrations of AHAs and BHAs that occur in commercial skin-food topicals are not nearly at the same level as prescription-strength products available through dermatologists. Be guided by your cosmetic dermatologist on the value of high-strength hydroxyl acid peels.

Fish Cartilage and Hyaluronic Acid

In 1992, researchers from the Helsinki Research Center in Finland showed that the topical application of ocean-fish cartilage can improve skin tone and decrease wrinkles (versus placebo) in healthy adult women. In more recent years, researchers have discovered that components found in fish cartilage can significantly inhibit the MMP enzymes that otherwise tear down collagen. Clinical studies show that fish-cartilage extracts are rich in GAGs that can improve the firmness of skin and its overall tone, and even reduce dark circles around the eyes.

The most important of these GAGs is almost certainly hyaluronic acid. It can bind more than one thousand times its weight in water and helps to provide volume and hydration to the skin. The absorption of hyaluronic acid into the skin has been documented, and indeed it may help carry other cosmetic ingredients. Reductions in the level of hyaluronic acid found in the skin through the aging process are thought to account for much of the wrinkling and loss of hydration and elasticity. Many topical formulas contain hyaluronic acid in its salt form, which is called sodium hyaluronate on the product label.

Soybeans

The topical application of soy extracts is a recent phenomenon, growing in large part thanks to two important studies in 2004. The first showed that topical soy milk reduced the risk of UV-induced skin cancer in animals. The second, a human study published in the *Journal of Cosmetic*

Science, showed that a fermented soy-milk extract with the antioxidant soy-derived chemicals genistein and daidzein improved skin elasticity after three months. Soy extracts can improve the production of the GAGs that support firm skin in a well-organized dermis. Follow-up studies have shown that, when topically applied, extracts of the fibrous germ layer in the coat of the soybean can reduce inflammation and protect against UV damage.

Research involving soy extracts for skin health continues. Most notably, research has shown that topical soy extracts keep the skin well hydrated by reinforcing epidermal skin-barrier function, improve the uniform color of aging skin (its tone), and decrease skin roughness and the appearance of fine lines and wrinkles. In addition, soy's anti-inflammatory properties against collagen-destroying PGE2 chemical have been reported, along with its ability to help with ongoing DNA repair in skin cells. In less than five years, soy extracts have established themselves as an important topical skin food.

TOMATOES AND SEAWEED

When we were researching the high-end cosmetic formulas of the 1950s, we were surprised to see creams with tomato and seaweed extracts. While there were some hints that chemicals within seaweed might stimulate collagen production, and tomatoes were known to contain vitamins A and C, no obvious research sixty years ago justified the inclusion of these two ingredients. Formulators were doing so based on intuition and traditional use.

Tomato extract contains collagen-protecting lycopene, and seaweeds contain a host of antioxidant and anti-inflammatory chemicals such as fucose and the omega-3 EPA.

In recent years, a polysaccharide chemical called fucose, which stimulates the production of the dermal scaffolding GAGs, has also been found in seaweed. In 2009, European researchers reported that seaweed fucose can inhibit the actions of AGEs in the skin. A study by French researchers in *Skin Research and Technology* (2005) showed that the topical application of fucose can significantly improve eye wrinkles in adult women after four weeks of use. The cream significantly improved parameters associated with wrinkle length and width in 65 percent of the cases.

Application of brown-seaweed extract protects against UV damage, reduces skin inflammation, and lowers oxidative stress. Specific brown seaweed used in Asian cuisine, *Undaria pinnatifida*, is emerging as the most skin-friendly seaweed because of its high content of anti-inflammatory omega-3 fatty acids.

Given its rich lycopene content, tomato extract seems like a very reasonable choice as a topical agent for skin protection. As discussed, lycopene is a key antioxidant in the skin. After UV exposure, the reserve levels of lycopene drop significantly due to its being called up to the front lines in defense. Topical lycopene can reduce inflammation and protect skin cells against UV damage and the thickening of the outer epidermis that otherwise occurs with UV exposure. In a human study, researchers from Italy showed that the topical application of lycopene gel outperformed a gel containing vitamins C and E in UV protection. It didn't take a whole lot of lycopene to provide protection against UV damage—the gel only contained 0.03 percent lycopene! Skin cream with tomato extract and seaweed? Great call.

Broccoli Extract

Broccoli undoubtedly is going to be the hottest topical skin food in the coming years. Researchers from Johns Hopkins have been investigating the properties of chemicals in broccoli for decades, mostly in the area of detoxification and cancer protection. One broccoli chemical in particular, sulforaphane, has emerged as the key agent that helps the body detoxify potential cancer-causing chemicals and associated free radicals. Researchers have shown that sulforaphane turns on what are called "Phase II" enzymes that make toxins more water soluble for removal.

When we think of detoxification, we tend to think about the liver, a clearinghouse where toxins are made more water soluble by Phase II enzymes for disposal via urine or bile. Yet what is often overlooked is that the liver is not the only place where Phase II detoxification is going on. These enzymes are active everywhere, including the skin.

Researchers from Johns Hopkins first showed that a topical, sulforaphane-rich broccoli extract could increase the activity of Phase II enzymes by more than fourfold in the skin of volunteers. Then, in a well-publicized study in the *Proceedings of the National Academy of Sciences* (2007), the researchers showed that the broccoli-sprout extract with sulforaphane could reduce UV-induced skin redness and inflammation by an average 38 percent in otherwise healthy adults.

Sulforaphane occurs naturally in a variety of the Brassica family vegetables that we recommended for youthful skin from the inside out on page 94. As soon as the researchers figure out how to get the green tint out of the broccoli extract while leaving in the important chemicals, you can be assured a new topical food for skin will be born. In the meantime, an extract of willow (Salix caprea), which has been shown to turn on the Phase II enzymes and protect against skin cancer, is starting to show up in topical anti-aging preparations.

AIR POLLUTION AND WIND

Sun exposure has been well established to accelerate the skin-aging process, yet other environmental assaults to the skin add to the vicious attack. In the early 1960s, researchers were reporting that pollution might be an underestimated factor in the acceleration of skin aging. In 1965, Pfizer launched a three-product topical cosmetic line called Beauty-Climate, with marketing materials stating, "Now we know. The greatest enemy of your complexion beauty isn't time. It's exposure. The city grime. Polluted air. Smog. Sun."

Perhaps this was a product before its time. Despite the big-dollar launch, the hoopla, and the full-page ads in best-selling magazines, Beauty-Climate, the promise of a cosmetic "that actually shelters your complexion" didn't stand the test of time. Yet, the premise of the product was quite accurate, and indeed more modern research has shown that air pollution does play a role.

Consider that when the primary chemical in air pollution, ozone, is exposed to skin, it can deplete antioxidant vitamins in the epidermis. To illustrate this, researchers from the University of California exposed mice to ozone-polluted air for two hours. Turns out that the polluted air caused a massive tenfold increase in oxidative stress within the skin, and the free-radical generation coincided with a 55 percent reduction in vitamin C levels and a 22 percent reduction in vitamin E levels within the skin.

Wind also appears to be an irritating factor in the skin-aging process, with one older study in the *British Journal of Dermatology* (1977) showing that laboratory animals exposed to wind and UV radiation were much more likely to develop skin cancer than those exposed to UV rays alone. While wind acts as a direct physical stressor to the skin, it may also carry pollutants to the skin surface. Hopefully researchers will revisit the wind and skin-aging connection with more detailed study.

Blood Orange

Varieties of red oranges that show up in North American supermarkets in the spring are especially high in a full complement of antioxidants, including the skin-friendly anthocyanins. Remember that the anthocyanins are the colorful, collagen-defending red-purple pigments found in fruits and berries. Red oranges also contain two other key antioxidants for the skin—caffeic and ferulic acids. Red oranges can protect against UV damage, with red-orange extract outperforming vitamin E in its ability to reduce sunburn and provide antioxidant support to the skin after UV exposure.

Interestingly, the topical application of caffeic acid has been shown to reduce the levels of collagen-damaging PGE2 in experimental animals after UV exposure. Caffeic acid, as its name hints, is also found in coffee. Perhaps it is no coincidence that coffee consumption has been shown to protect against skin cancer in a number of large population studies. The other natural chemical in red oranges, ferulic acid, has also been shown to act synergistically with vitamins C and E to protect against UV-induced skin cell damage in human studies. Undoubtedly, the many natural chemical offerings of red-orange extract make it a suitable candidate to feed the skin externally.

TOPICAL ANTIOXIDANTS ENHANCE MAINSTREAM DERMATOLOGICAL CARE

Skilled cosmetic dermatologists employ cutting-edge techniques from botox to lasers, all of which can make a difference in the maintenance of youthful, glowing skin. It is important to note that feeding the skin with oral and topical nutrients is not mutually exclusive from the interventions commonly used by mainstream dermatology.

A study in the *Journal of Dermatological Treatment* (2008) highlights the adjunctive value of topical skin nutrition. In this case, the topical application of a plant-based antioxidant blend plus microdermabrasion significantly improved a variety of objective skin-aging measurements, including dermal thickness, more than treatment with microdermabrasion alone. Separate research has shown that combining antioxidants with prescription glycolic acid provides a synergistic effect in the skin.

Ginger and Turmeric

Since both of these roots have so much to offer as internal skin protectants, it shouldn't be surprising that researchers have been investigating their topical use as well. Both ginger and turmeric have a long history of being added to oil and applied topically for the promotion of healthy skin or wound repair in South Asia. Knowing what we now know about the ability of certain polyunsaturated fats to carry food-based chemicals through the skin layers via their pull-and-drag properties, there seems to have been some wisdom in using oils to massage small amounts of the mashed or powdered root into the skin.

While the key anti-inflammatory chemicals in ginger (gingerols) appear to perfuse through the skin quite well, turmeric's principal antioxidant and UV-protecting chemical, curcumin, needs help to get through the skin. The EPA from fish oil might be just the ticket to help access the deeper skin layers.

The anti-inflammatory and antioxidant properties of curcumin and the gingerols after topical application are becoming more apparent with each passing month. Recently, an extract from Asian turmeric was shown to promote collagen production and decrease collagen-destroying MMPs in a more effective manner than green-tea antioxidants. Chemicals from both roots have protected the skin against UV damage in experimental studies.

A study in the *International Journal of Dermatology* (2006) showed that a topical ginger extract inhibited wrinkle formation in animals exposed to chronic, yet only low-level UV radiation over three months. The researchers set it up that way on purpose so that the low-level UV rays did not cause the usual redness and acute sunburn in the animals—this to reflect the day-to-day UV exposure of most humans. Incredibly, the ginger extract maintained the normal elasticity of the skin and prevented wrinkles despite the chronic UV exposure. Indeed, the ginger extract inhibited the enzyme that breaks down the elastic fibers (elastase), and the natural structure of the dermal elastic fibers was maintained.

Interestingly, the same researchers also applied a synthetic topical UV sunscreen, and while it may protect against sunburn, it did not protect the elastic fibers and did not prevent wrinkling. Again, we are not saying that sunscreens are of no value. They are, yet we should not rely upon them as the sole means to stop the aging process. Doing so might set you up for disappointment.

Most studies on the topical application of ginger and turmeric are only in the experimental stages, so at the time of this writing, human data is still lacking. All we have at the moment is one human study that used a 0.1 percent curcumin formula along with other herbs. In that study, published in *Phytomedicine* (2007), the combination herbal formula with curcumin improved skin firmness and elasticity after four weeks.

New ginger extracts that have some of the skin irritants removed are in the development phase and will be in commercial use shortly. This is an important development because ginger has some fat-soluble components that can irritate the skin and cause undesirable flushing.

Cocoa

With the exciting studies showing that oral ingestion of 329 milligrams of cocoa antioxidants improves blood flow to the skin, enhances hydration, increases dermal thickness, and decreases roughness and scaling, cocoa is the new "it" ingredient for skin. At this point, we are not entirely sure that the benefits obtained via internal consumption of cocoa antioxidants will translate into a new topical skin food. However, the early research indicators are good.

In a landmark study published in the *International Journal of Cosmetic Science* (2008), researchers from Belgium (of course!) showed that the cocoa antioxidants improved GAG production and turned on collagen formation in human skin cells. Once again, not much cocoa extract was needed get the job done. The researchers figured that between 0.5 and 0.75 percent cocoa antioxidants was the optimal topical dose. The good news for any fan of topical cocoa butter is that the researchers also reported that the cocoa antioxidants work better in helping to maintain a youthful skin structure when delivered in a cocoa-butter base.

Taking it a step further, the researchers compared the cocoa antioxidants to an expensive anti-aging topical and found that it was "comparable (or better, in the case of collagen I) than a commercially available anti-ageing cream." Also in 2007, researchers showed in experimental studies that topical cocoa extracts can prevent UV-induced collagen destruction and wrinkle formation. The stock of cocoa extract as a topical skin food is definitely rising.

Tea and Wine

While green tea gets all the attention, the entire tea family should be considered a friend to the skin. The idea of topical tea for the skin is certainly not a new one. Placing cooled, wet tea bags over the eyes has been going on as long as tea has been held in some sort of bag. The explosion in the interest of tea as an external skin food was spurred by Japanese studies in the 1980s that showed green-tea application might help prevent skin cancer.

Virtually all teas (with various degrees of fermentation) derived from the *Camellia sinensis* tea plant—white, green, oolong, and black teas—have been shown to protect against UV damage, decrease inflammation, and lower oxidative stress in skin cells under experimental settings. Another unrelated tea, the red rooibos tea from South Africa, has also been shown to inhibit skin cancer in animals when applied topically.

Most of the data on the anti-aging properties of topical tea extracts have been confined to animal studies, although one recent study showed that topical tea extracts (green and black teas) can reduce inflammation and restore the integrity of the skin in cancer patients undergoing radiation. Topical green and other teas are probably best combined with other antioxidants, as highlighted by a study in the *Journal of Drugs in Dermatology* (2007), which showed that topical green and white tea, along with pomegranate and mangosteen fruit, improved the overall appearance and texture of facial skin among healthy middle-aged women.

RED WINE AND UV PROTECTION

In a well-publicized study appearing in the *Journal of the German Society of Dermatology* (2009), researchers reported that oral consumption of red wine, which is high in naturally occurring antioxidants, can protect against UV-induced sunburn. This was yet another indicator that internal nutrition and the inside-out delivery of antioxidant and anti-inflammatory chemicals can influence the externally visible signs of aging.

Some of the chemicals within wine may indeed protect against UV damage when topically applied. One such red-wine chemical, resveratrol, has been shown in experimental settings to reduce UV-induced skin-cell damage. Another chemical from the seeds of grapes has been shown to have wound-healing properties and to protect against UV damage when applied topically.

Japanese researchers have been investigating sake (rice wine) as a skin food for a number of years. As reported by one expert from Gifu University in Japan, the Japanese have used sake as a skin-care lotion since ancient times, and women who live in the northern regions where sake consumption is high tend to have a smoother complexion and skin condition. The initial scientific studies have shown that topical application or oral consumption of sake can help maintain epidermal barrier integrity after UV exposure.

Some of the chemicals derived from rice wine have been shown to stimulate production of the lipids that make up the mortar of the epidermal brick wall. According to a 2009 study by Korean researchers, the benefits of topical sake extracts extend down further than the epidermis. The researchers found that sake stimulated collagen production, decreased inflammation, and slowed down the collagen-destroying MMPs. With sake possessing all of these skin-friendly properties, it is no wonder that a 2 percent topical sake extract prevented dehydration and skin wrinkling with chronic low-grade UV exposure over time. Based on the results so far and the long history of sake use in Japan, we are confident that sake extracts will soon be a new topical skin food for North Americans.

Botanical Odds 'n' Ends

In 2007 to 2009, a number of studies were published on a variety of herbal ingredients used as topical anti-aging and UV-protecting agents. Let's take a moment to discuss some botanicals that have either started to—or are destined to—show up in natural skin preparations.

HORSE CHESTNUT EXTRACT

Japanese researchers reported in the *International Journal of Cosmetic Science* (2007) that applying a 3 percent horse chestnut extract topically for nine weeks significantly decreased wrinkle scores (versus the control) in otherwise healthy women. Horse chestnut has a long history of use as a botanical that improves blood flow, and research has shown it possesses strong antioxidant and anti-inflammatory activities. The experimental studies leading up to the clinical trial suggested that horse chestnut extract can improve elasticity of the skin.

GOTU KOLA (*CENTELLA ASIATICA*)

Gotu kola (*Centella asiatica*) is another botanical that can improve blood flow—and one rich in antioxidant and anti-inflammatory chemicals. In Asian nations the herb has a long history of use in skin care, particularly for wound healing. Recently researchers have discovered that one of the chemicals in gotu kola, called asiaticoside, can stimulate collagen production. In another study published again in the *International Journal of Cosmetic Science* (2008), researchers showed that a cream containing just 0.1 percent asiaticoside significantly improved eye wrinkles, skin pigmentation, elasticity, roughness, and hydration. Evaluation with instrumentation confirmed that the asiaticoside cream decreased the depths of wrinkles after three months.

BURDOCK ROOT (*ARCTIUM LAPPA*)

Burdock root (*Arctium lappa*) is part of the traditional Japanese diet, and you can see it for sale in most Japanese grocery stores, where it is usually called gobo. It, too, has a long history of use for skin conditions, particularly inflammatory ones such as psoriasis, acne, and eczema. Researchers from Germany identified the component of burdock with the highest anti-inflammatory activity, a chemical called arctiin, and subsequently determined that it stimulated collagen production. In a study published in the *Journal of Cosmetic Science* (2008), a topical burdock extract with 0.25 percent arctiin was shown to increase collagen production and GAGs, improve hydration, and significantly reduce facial wrinkling, compared to the control group. The impressive results were noted between one to three months of regular use.

BILBERRY

Bilberry, also known as the European blueberry, has a long history of use in skin care. Among the blueberry species, bilberry is incredibly rich in colorful antioxidants called anthocyanins that can protect the integrity of collagen. Experimental studies have shown that the purple anthocyanins found in bilberry can protect against UV damage by inhibiting the MMPs involved in collagen destruction. Antioxidants derived from berries within the blueberry family have been shown to inhibit glycation in the skin. In addition, oil derived from bilberry has been shown to improve skin hydration and the overall texture of the skin.

EVEN MORE...

Honorable mentions go out to pomegranate, rosemary, licorice, ginseng, feverfew, and milk thistle extracts, which have recently been shown to have anti-inflammatory and antioxidant activity in skin cells. In addition, experimental studies show that saffron, Indian gooseberry, and green coffee-bean oil can stimulate collagen and GAG production in experimental settings. All of these botanicals are currently the subject of intense research, and a variety of patents are being issued for the extracts in aspects of skin care.

Some of the research has shown a specific ability to reduce UV-induced oxidative stress. Milk thistle, which is traditionally used as a liver-detoxifying botanical, has been shown in human research to improve rosacea when topically applied. Some of these ingredients, or chemicals derived from these herbs, are now showing up in anti-aging skin-care creams.

Topical Application

It is important to remember that the application of raw herbs may on occasion do the skin more harm than good. Any skin-care company worth its salt will do extensive research and due diligence in determining if the herbs may induce skin sensitivities. Feverfew provides a perfect example because it is well known to cause skin irritation when applied topically, or even touched by gardeners. That didn't stop the scientists at Johnson & Johnson who devoted years of research and development to develop a topical feverfew extract that works—yet without the skin irritant called parthenolide. Parthenolide-depleted feverfew protects against UV-induced sunburn in adults and lowers oxidative stress while protecting DNA in the skin.

Another example is ginger extract, which needs to have lipid soluble components removed to prevent skin irritation. The point is that despite the massive potential of botanical medicine in topical anti-aging skin care, there are some risks. The onus is on companies to do their homework and provide effective products with ingredients and extracts that will only serve to improve the appearance of your skin, not make it worse.

CONTROVERSY: DO SUNSCREENS PROTECT AGAINST SKIN MELANOMA?

Fact: No solid evidence shows that sunscreens protect against melanoma, the deadliest of skin cancers. In eighteen pooled studies, researchers could find no evidence of this type of protection. At least one study has shown a *higher* risk of melanoma in users of sunscreens. There are a number of possible reasons for this, including the false sense of security provided by sunscreens.

In a famous study by dermatology researchers at the University of Texas, those beachgoers who used the highest SPF sunscreens paradoxically had a higher frequency of sunburn and spent longer hours in the sun during peak hours. Research also shows that those who apply sunscreens in real-life settings, such as on the beach, are not likely to do so with the accurate laboratory techniques that were used in establishing the SPF number. In other words, we typically don't do a good job with sunscreen application.

The plot thickens a little when you consider that a few studies have shown that sunscreen application can actually increase oxidative stress in the skin. As reported in *Free Radical Biology & Medicine* (2006), the initial application of sunscreen can limit free-radical generation in the skin. However, an hour after application, the pendulum swings the other way, and there is an increase in free radical generation in the epidermis, well beyond that with UV exposure alone.

Up to 2 percent of some of the synthetic chemicals in sunscreens are making it into body-wide circulation and even into breast milk. The health implications of this are unknown, and at the time of this writing, some companies are developing sunscreens based on organic ingredients only. We are certainly not suggesting abandonment of sunscreens. The protective influence in non-melanoma skin cancers has been established, and proper use is advised for this reason.

Royal Jelly: Told You So

Royal jelly is the food delivered to the queen bee by the worker bees; it is reserved for the queen alone. As mentioned earlier, royal jelly was a hot item in the high-end skin creams of the mid-1950s when it came on the topical skin-care scene. The marketers, some of whom referred to royal jelly in ads as "the secret to eternal youth," really didn't know why they were promoting it in a scientific sense, although there was awareness of its fatty acids and they did discuss it as being a nutrient-rich food for the skin.

Yet the "experts" laughed it off as useless, and since the big players in the commercial skin-care industry are always looking for the next "big" thing, royal jelly faded away—only to be replaced by other ingredients that were, in all reality, probably less effective.

Vindication for the use of royal jelly as a topical anti-aging ingredient would come in 2004 when researchers from the famed Fujisaki Institute in Japan took a fresh look at it. In published research, they determined that royal jelly does indeed have collagen-stimulating properties. Specifically, it was determined that the fatty acids within the royal jelly are the potent stimulators of collagen production.

The researchers proved that royal jelly's fatty acids turn on a specific chemical involved in the early stages of collagen production. Interestingly, one of the key collagen-stimulating chemicals in royal jelly is structurally similar to glycolic acid, the known collagen stimulator we discussed in the alpha-hydroxy acid section. The Japanese scientists didn't discover that royal jelly is the secret to eternal youth. However, they certainly justified its (or its fatty acids') inclusion in skin creams.

Energizing Your Skin Cells

As we discussed in chapter 6, the condition of our skin through the aging process is only as good as the strength and efficiency of the mitochondria in our skin cells. During the aging process, the mitochondrial efficiency diminishes, and with decreased efficiency comes the generation of free radicals from the skin cell itself. In other words, mitochondria that start to become inefficient will become the actual source of oxidative stress and damaging inflammatory chemicals.

You can imagine aged mitochondria as an old leaky, crusted battery that is struggling to provide your skin cells with the energy to function. The good news is that internal nutrition can both protect our mitochondria and increase its efficiency. Emerging science is showing that we can also feed the mitochondria from the outside in.

CoQ_{10} is perhaps the best-known supporter of mitochondrial function in the skin-care world. Although we are capable of manufacturing our own CoQ_{10} in the body, our ability to do so weakens with the passage of time. Research has established that our skin levels of CoQ_{10} diminish through the aging process, just when we need it most. Skin CoQ_{10} levels also drop when we are faced with UV radiation—almost certainly because the CoQ_{10} is being used up in the defensive struggle to protect us.

In a landmark study published in the journal *Biofactors* (2008), German researchers showed that skin cells from older adults (ages sixty-one to seventy-three) are struggling to get energy produced. Compared to skin cells from young adults (ages nineteen to thirty-seven), the older group were burning through 30 percent more sugar to get the energy necessary for skin-cell function. This certainly highlights the loss of efficiency in our skin cells. What made this a stand-out study was that the topical application of just 0.01 percent CoQ$_{10}$ (twice daily for seven days) significantly improved the functioning of the mitochondria.

In another study in *Biofactors* (2008), Japanese researchers showed that a 1 percent CoQ$_{10}$ cream significantly improved wrinkle scores (versus cream with no CoQ$_{10}$) after three months. Most of the studies on CoQ$_{10}$ had focused on its ability to protect against UV damage and to turn down the dial on the enzymes that break down collagen. The emerging research suggests that its ability to recharge the skin batteries may be its most important attribute.

CoQ$_{10}$ is not the only topical battery charger; the topical application of α-lipoic acid is also capable of supporting the mitochondria through the aging process. In fact, α-lipoic acid penetrates well through the epidermis and into the dermal layers where its antioxidant and anti-inflammatory properties provide a protective edge. In a study published in the *British Journal of Dermatology* (2003), researchers reported that a 5 percent α-lipoic acid cream applied twice daily for three months improved skin roughness, overall tone, and the appearance of fine lines.

Another well-known mitochondria supporter is creatine. Yet it was ignored as a topical ingredient until 2005 when German researchers reported for the first time that it could protect against UV-induced oxidative stress and aging. Creatine permeates through the skin quite well and reaches the dermal layers. In human research, it has been shown to significantly improve the structure of the epidermal-dermal junction after four weeks of topical application.

Recall that the epidermal-dermal junction flattens out through the aging process and blood flow to the area is compromised. Creatine appeared to reverse this trend. Researchers, who decided to try a combination of CoQ$_{10}$ and creatine, found that when it was applied for three months, there was a significant improvement in wrinkle reduction and skin elasticity versus with

CoQ_{10} alone. In a study published in the *Journal of Cosmetic Dermatology* (2008), researchers also showed that a combination of topical folic acid and creatine improved skin firmness and roughness, and decreased wrinkle volume in middle-aged adults after four weeks.

Other mitochondrial supporters include the botanicals rhodiola and ginkgo, grape skin extracts with resveratrol, as well as the antioxidant flavonoid quercetin. Mitochondria have only recently been shown to accumulate large amounts of quercetin. They are even more apt to do so when inflammation and oxidative stress start to elevate. Until 2009, researchers had assumed that quercetin protects mitochondria from the outside, not realizing that our skin cells sequester quercetin during times of need. Experimental research shows that topical quercetin protects against UV-induced oxidative stress and helps to preserve glutathione, one of the skin's most important antioxidants.

Rhodiola and ginkgo can protect skin cells under stress when applied topically. Indeed, rhodiola has been combined recently with a topical AGE-inhibitor called L-carnosine and shown to improve the skin-barrier function in adults with sensitive skin.

A new wave of natural, topical skin-care products will undoubtedly focus on both mitochondrial stimulation and AGE inhibition. Curcumin from turmeric, ginger, quercetin, the amino acid L-carnosine, green tea, and other AGE-inhibitors will be well suited to join mitochondrial battery chargers in promoting youthful skin by natural means.

Topical Probiotics

For centuries, fermented milk products have been used as a topical method of rejuvenating the skin. As mentioned earlier, European dermatologist Jaime Peyri reported in the *Journal of Cutaneous Diseases* (1912) that freshly prepared topical *Lactobacillus bulgaricus* was helpful for acne and skin inflammation.

Under the modern scientific eye, the benefits of doing so have been largely attributed to the alpha-hydroxy acids (AHAs) in fermented dairy. However, a study in the *Journal of Investigative Dermatology* (1999) suggested that there may be more to it. Perhaps the friendly bacteria in fermented dairy were contributing to the promotion of healthy skin. Specifically, the researchers found that a strain of friendly bacteria (*Streptococcus*), one used to make most commercial yogurts, increased production of ceramides. As you may remember, ceramides make up the mortar in the brick-and-mortar wall of the epidermis. The integrity of the ceramide mortar is essential in keeping the skin well hydrated because ceramide levels drop through the aging process— and when ceramide levels drop, inflammation in the skin increases.

Looking more closely, researchers found that the probiotic bacterium contains enzymes that support the production of certain fatty components of ceramides. In the ten years since the discovery, studies have shown that the topical application of S. *thermophilus* can improve hydration and decrease inflammation in patients with chronic dermatitis.

Other researchers reported in the *International Wound Journal* (2009) that a *Lactobacillus plantarum* probiotic, freshly prepared and applied daily for ten days, was as effective in the promotion of wound healing as the conventionally applied drug (silver sulphadiazine). The *Lactobacillus* probiotic used in the study has been shown to lower inflammation, dampening the same inflammatory fires that otherwise destroy collagen. The probiotic also inhibits the growth of undesirable bacteria that can otherwise turn on enzymes that will break down the structural components of your dermis. Korean researchers also reported that probiotic *Lactococcus* can secrete chemicals that prevent the growth of undesirable bacteria that would otherwise cause inflammation in the skin. Another blossoming area of research is the use of probiotic bacteria to ferment botanical ingredients before they are added to skin-care products. It has been shown that fermentation may improve the collagen and dermal boosting activity of herbal ingredients. For example, a study in the *Journal of Ethnopharmacology* (2009) showed that probiotic-fermented astragalus (Asian herb traditionally used for energy support) boosted hyaluronic acid GAG production far more than the unfermented herb. Lactobacillus-fermented herbs may have greater anti-inflammatory properties and enhanced absorption in the skin.

Since probiotic bacteria have antioxidant, anti-inflammatory, and anti-microbial activity, they represent a strong addition to the natural topical arsenal in the defense of youthful skin. In addition, acid secreted by live probiotics can help maintain the "acid mantle" of the skin. The surface pH of the skin is normally in the acid range, and alterations due to the use of alkaline soaps and hard alkaline water have been associated with chronic inflammation of the skin. The maintenance of an acidic outer-skin surface is unrelated to, and should not be confused with, the overwhelmingly, unhealthy acidic diet we have discussed (see page 157). Certain locations in the body—the gut and the skin—should be quite acidic due to secretions of much-needed friendly bacteria.

Given the great potential of probiotics, it is clear to see why a number of commercial cosmetic companies are racing to get in on the bacterial act. Yet aside from *S. thermophilus* and a few other strains, topical probiotics and their potential in skin-care are not well known. Virtually nothing is known, for example, about the ability of probiotics to function after unrefrigerated storage in a container full of cosmetic chemicals. And you can't rub any old refrigerated yogurt on your body and expect it to work, either. The sugar content of most commercial yogurts would undo any potential benefit of the bacteria, assuming the yogurt even contained live, active cultures.

Many of the key benefits of probiotics are only due to their ability to produce and secrete chemicals that have anti-microbial effects, act as antioxidants, and so on. Therefore, if the new waves of topical probiotic potions contain only dead bacteria, and that is very likely, the potential benefit to the skin will be very limited indeed. Certain heat-killed probiotics may stimulate the immune system in a beneficial way. For example, a new study in the journal *Experimental Dermatology* (2009) shows that nonliving Bifidobacterium longum (topically applied probiotic) can reduce skin reactions and improve hydration in adults with sensitive skin. On the flip side, the nasty bacteria that can contribute to acne, Propionibacterium acnes, has recently been shown to induce inflammation in the skin even when it has been heat-killed. However, the vast majority of benefits are derived from living probiotics and the chemicals they secrete while alive.

Two key words are associated with the historical use and recent 2009 study on wound repair with *Lactobacillus* cultures—freshly prepared. In our opinion, when probiotics are stored on shelves in cosmetic formulas, the cart is going before the scientific horse. Aside from the heat of transport and shelf-storage, many of the chemicals within cosmetic formulations will cause the probiotics to die off. While the fermentation of herbs by probiotic bacteria may enhance absorption and bioavailability of some of the chemicals within plants (before the packaging stage), certain botanical ingredients can interfere with the shelf life of probiotics. That said, a glimmer of hope still shines for the emergence of legitimate probiotic incorporation into cosmetics.

A technique called microencapsulation can coat the bacteria and allow them to live at room temperature unencumbered by the presence of oil-based ingredients. The microencapsulated probiotic bacteria can live within pure borage oil, omega-3 oils, and other members of the DermaLipid family of skin lipids (essential fatty acids, ceramides, phosphatidylserine, and squalene). The probiotics will not live long, even microencapsulated, in the presence of other non-lipid cosmetic ingredients.

Until further research proves otherwise and until stability issues are sorted out, a fresh, homemade probiotic paste is likely to provide far better results than the early entries into the topical realm. Natren, a reputable probiotic company, provides recipes for topical probiotic paste on its website, http://www.natren.com.

Good for You and the Environment

Many of the chemicals used in mass-marketed cosmetic formulas have toxicity risks associated with them, and some of these chemicals end up in our environment where they can continue to wreak havoc for decades. A number of recent books have tackled the subject of harmful cosmetics, and a full discussion of the almost ten thousand ingredients that show up in cosmetics is beyond the scope of this book.

Simply placing the words "natural" or "with natural ingredients" on a cosmetic label tells the consumer nothing about the true integrity of the finished product. It may still be surrounded by potentially harmful ingredients. Given the estimate that the average woman applies more that 150 cosmetic chemicals to the skin per day, more unknowns than knowns exist with such cosmetic combinations. Studies from Duke University have shown that the supposed safety of one topically applied synthetic chemical may disappear when it is combined with other synthetic chemicals.

The primary concerns are associated with cancer-causing chemicals, ingredients that can mimic or disturb human hormone levels in children, and ingredients that may cover up wrinkles yet ultimately accelerate the aging process. Many consumers are already aware of the concerns associated with parabens, sodium lauryl sulfate, and mineral oils. However, the ingredient list in mass-marketed cosmetics can get long, and consumers need a quick resource for guidance. Thankfully, the not-for-profit Environmental Working Group (EWG) has spent countless hours taking stock of virtually every ingredient that will show up in a cosmetic formula. The EWG provides a simple, no-cost summary of cosmetic ingredients based on a 0-to-10 hazard scale. Simply plug the name of any cosmetic ingredient into the Skin Deep search engine, and a summary will be provided covering the areas of cancer, allergies, reproductive risks, and others. The EWG website (http://www.ewg.org) is a go-to resource for all who are concerned about what they feed their skin day after day, night after night.

Another gold-standard resource is the section of the Whole Foods Market website devoted to the company's Premium Body Care standard. Whole Foods Market assembled experts who combed through the scientific data for two years before establishing a list of some 250 chemicals that are not permitted to be in the personal-care products that the company carries. The Whole Foods Market experts understood that some synthetic ingredients are necessary to act as preservatives and surfactants. They simply eliminated the ones deemed most likely to cause harm or to have gaps in safety data A quick trip to the Whole Foods Market site (http://www.wholefoodsmarket.com) for more information on the Premium Body Care standard is a no-cost venture that will certainly help guide you and your family in making decisions on chemical ingredients.

For too long, the cosmetics industry has been regulated like the Wild West, hiding behind a foil-thin badge of minimal oversight by the U.S. Food and Drug Administration (FDA). In reality, the FDA does not require cosmetics to be tested for safety before entering the marketplace, relying instead upon companies to substantiate the safety of the finished goods. With no mandatory testing, the politically influential industry is, in essence, regulating itself.

In fairness, many companies are responding to consumer demands, and there is certainly much more transparency among even the larger companies. Fewer and fewer companies are hiding cancer-causing chemicals behind a "trade-secret" loophole that allows chemicals to be listed as simply "fragrance." Today, wise consumers want to know exactly what the "fragrance" consists of, and an increasing number of consumers are turning their backs on products without full disclosure. What started as a grassroots effort has shifted policy among the big players.

Today, consumers also demand more than efficacy from companies that profess to have their interest at heart. They also want to know about the long-term generational aspects of the safety, sustainability, and overall environmental impact of the ingredients.

Not that long ago, the biggest players in the cosmetic industry hunted the globe for "the world's costliest ingredients" (including turtle and shark) and bragged about it. Not only is this now passé, but for many wise consumers of today, it is also a complete turnoff. Consumers want ingredients that are environmentally friendly and sustainable. They want ingredients that will not enter the bloodstream and act as hormone disrupters, and will not be cancer-causing agents in themselves or their grandchildren. Consumers are demanding that companies take responsibility for synthetic ingredients that are known to bio-accumulate and persist in our wildlife and our environment at large.

Cause for Concern

A recent study in the *Journal of Investigative Dermatology* (2008) sent shock waves through the industry and clearly highlights the massive gap in the safety research of mass-marketed products. Very little research has been conducted on what happens when mass-market moisturizing creams and lotions are applied topically *after* UV exposure. Sure, we know a fair bit about blocking the effects of UV with topicals, but what happens when moisturizers are added afterwards? It turns out that a number of commercially available moisturizers can *increase* the risk of skin cancer in animals that had been exposed to the UV radiation—and not just by a little bit.

Researchers found that the number of skin tumors after topical moisturizer increased by 79 percent. As the researchers stated in the study, "Skin-care preparations are generally not tested for carcinogenic activity per se or for carcinogenic activity in animals previously exposed chronically to UVB." The good news is that when Johnson & Johnson prepared a custom moisturizer for the same researchers that contained no sodium lauryl sulfate, mineral oil, petrolatum, or any paraben-based ingredients, there was no increase in tumor risk. Obviously lots of work is required to sort this out.

More disconcerting evidence on sunscreen ingredients is highlighted by a study in *Free Radical Biology & Medicine* (2006), which showed an important downside to some topically applied chemicals. While the UV sunscreens worked well initially and kept oxidative stress in check, the pendulum swung the other way after sixty minutes and the presence of the synthetic UV blockers actually *increased* free radical production.

When you combine this information with other research showing that UV blockers don't stop elastic fiber damage and wrinkling after chronic UV exposure, the time to consider the chemical composition of these blockers more closely has already passed. Suffice it to say that research is finally highlighting the potential dangers in our cosmetic cabinets.

STAY INDOORS WITH YOUR SUNLESS TAN

Sunless tanning sprays and lotions may seem like an attractive alternative. Just don't go out in the sun while wearing the fake tan. A 2008 study showed that chemicals within sunless tanning agents increase free-radical production in the skin and increase the risk of sun-induced damage within 24 hours of application.

SUNSCREEN QUANDARY

In 2008, the not-for-profit Environmental Working Group (EWG) looked at nearly one thousand name-brand sunscreens and found that only one in five provided the delicate balance between adequate UVA-B protection and the absence of chemicals that may do more harm than good. This, combined with research indicating that some synthetic sunscreens can increase UV-induced oxidative stress in the skin after one hour, leaves consumers in a quandary. Thankfully, the EWG folks provide guidance on the most effective and safe sunscreens to help protect you from cancer and keep your skin younger.

EWG's Top Sunscreen Picks

Blue Lizard

California Baby

CVS with Zinc Oxide

Jason Natural Cosmetics

Kiss My Face

Neutrogena Sensitive Skin

Olay Defense Daily UV Moisturizer

SkinCeuticals

Solar Sense

Walgreens Zinc Oxide

Check www.ewg.org to see if your sunscreen is among the 171 products that made the cut.

Marketing Hype

Looking back at the full-page marketing campaigns of the 1950s and 1960s, we found fashion magazines peppered with so-called and undisclosed youth ingredients discovered "behind the closed doors." One high-end product was trademarked, if you can believe it, as the *Cup of Youth*, and, given its name, it was packaged not in a standard jar, but in an actual goblet! The full page ad in *Vogue* for this Cup of Youth carried the tagline, "Since time began, women have searched for this!" with an additional promise that "The signs of age will melt away."

Thankfully, those days are over. Wise consumers are no longer seduced by the illusion that Ponce de Leon, PhD, is hard at work behind closed doors filling goblets with youth ingredients derived from some mystical fountain adjacent to the factory. Wise consumers are disinterested in testimonials and unpublished research that companies have "on file." Extensive research by BrandSpark International has shown that the top priority of today's skin-care consumer is finding products that have proven efficacy. Although price ranks high, scientific evidence of results remains in the poll position.

Some natural ingredients are hyped up for anti-aging properties—the berries from the coffee plant being a prime example—yet when you look closely, there aren't even any peer-reviewed published experimental studies to discuss, let alone human clinical trials. Companies that claim all sorts of amazing research, yet hold back that research from the critical scientific eye of peer review, will ultimately be punished by consumers. The hype rapidly fades away, much like the aforementioned *Cup of Youth*—both the goblet and the trademark have been abandoned by its manufacturer.

Wise consumers today have more realistic expectations. They know no goblet of youth exists; they simply want a product that will provide "real-world" results, such as a meaningful change in visible signs of aging, or an effective product that will noticeably support the skin and slow down the inevitable progression of the skin-aging process. There is no fountain of youth; there is no cup, goblet, or chalice of youth, but that doesn't mean we should sit idly by and let accelerated skin aging just happen. The published research described in this chapter shows us that a number of foods and botanical-based ingredients can feed the skin from the outside in. By doing so, they have the potential to improve hydration, act as a dent-remover and smooth out the skin to a noticeable degree, provide a degree of UV protection, and ultimately add a layer of insulation against the aging process.

PROCEED WITH CAUTION—THE CHEMICALS TO LOOK OUT FOR

The Environmental Working Group (EWG) and Whole Foods Market cosmetic experts have raised concerns about a number of ingredients. Here are some synthetic chemical groups that make up large families—some of these ingredients and their family members have been reported as potentially hazardous by the EWG or are banned for cosmetic use by Whole Foods Markets. For example, there are many steareths, and some have a better safety record and are more suitable in natural cosmetics than others. Simply check your cosmetic ingredients at http://www.cosmeticdatabase.com to get a gauge of the hazard score (1 to 10 scale) for specific cosmetic ingredients. To check out Whole Food Premium Body Care banned chemical list, visit www.wholefoodsmarket.com.

- Acetamide MEA
- Aluminums
- Ammoniums
- BHA and BHT
- Ceramides (synthetic)
- Ceteareths
- Cocamides
- Dimethylamine
- EDTA
- Hydroxypropyl
- Isopropyls
- Laureth-7
- Mineral oil
- Myristyls
- Oleths
- Parabens
- PEGs
- Petrolatum
- Polyglyceryls
- Propylene glycol
- Simethicone
- Sodium laureth sulfate
- Steareths

LAVENDER CAVEAT

Due to its anti-inflammatory activity, lavender has become a primary ingredient in a number of commercially available topical formulas. However, a study in the journal *Cell Proliferation* (2004) showed that higher concentrations of lavender may actually damage skin fibroblasts, the cells that make collagen.

In addition, research published in the *New England Journal of Medicine* (2007) hints that lavender may cause the growth of breast tissue in young boys. The condition, known as gyneco-mastia, resolved itself when the lavender was discontinued. While we are not concerned with the tiny amounts of lavender used as a fragrance in natural skin foods, its use as a primary medicinal ingredient for skin remains a concern. Be wary when you see lavender at the top of an ingredient list.

BEST INGREDIENTS TO FEED THE SKIN

- α-lipoic acid
- Anthocyanins and proanthocyanins from bilberry, grapes, and red-purple foods
- B vitamins—including B2, 3, 6, and 12 and folic acid
- Ceramides from wheat germ or rice bran
- Cocoa
- CoQ_{10}
- Creatine
- Curcumin
- EPA from deodorized fish oil
- Fish collagen peptides
- GLA from borage and/or evening primrose oil
- Horse chestnut and burdock
- Olive, sesame, and rice-bran oils
- Phosphatidylserine
- Royal jelly
- Seaweed
- Soy extracts
- Squalene from plant source
- Tea extracts—white, oolong, green
- Tomato extract with lycopene
- Vitamin A retinol
- Vitamin C ester
- Vitamin E ester

8

Dietary Plan of Action and Recipes

Key Dietary Notes

- The first priority is to color the plate as much as possible. Consume a minimum of five servings of *deeply colored* vegetables and fruits—note the deeply colored part of the equation.
- Include fish at least five times per week, and choose oily, low mercury fish (such as wild salmon, sardines, anchovies, and mackerel). If you can't commit to the oily fish, supplementation becomes a priority.
- Choose complex, fiber-rich carbohydrates—brown rice, whole-wheat pasta, whole-grain cereals, whole-grain breads—instead of their white, refined, and bleached counterparts.
- Avoid corn, safflower, sunflower, and soybean oils while cooking and in purchased foods. Look out for them in prepared foods such as baked goods and salad dressings. Cook with organic canola oil and extra-virgin olive oil. Rice bran and sesame oils are rich sources of antioxidants and can also be alternated with olive and canola oils in cooking and salads. Avoid margarine and butter.
- Limit intake of high-AGE foods (fatty meats cooked on high and dry heat, full-fat cheeses, highly processed foods, and dry baked goods cooked on high heat). These foods promote oxidative stress and inflammation, and compromise the long-term health of collagen.

The general rule is to limit AGE with a lower cooking temperature, less cooking time, and increased moisture.

- Include culinary spices and herbs, and moderate teas and coffee to provide anti-inflammatory and antioxidant protection for the skin.

- Take a daily multivitamin, probiotic, and fish oil and, unless you feel very confident in your adherence to the first priority above (the vegetable and fruits), include a powdered super-food formula.

About the Recipes

The following meal ideas should serve as a reminder to steam, boil, stew, simmer, and poach as much as possible. Firing up the oven and cooking at 400°F is the nutritional equivalent of pulling out an old-school sunlamp and baking yourself in front of it. Just as surely as some types of foods can protect against the visible signs of aging, some cooking techniques will promote oxidative stress, inflammation, alterations to the friendly gut bacteria, collagen destruction, and ultimately wrinkles. Any dietary plan for the prevention of the visible signs of aging that does not take into consideration the Advanced Glycation End-products (AGEs) in foods is an incomplete plan.

Foods cooked on high heat in the absence of water—think ovens, grills, and skillets—promote oxidative stress, free radicals, and inflammation in consumers of such foods. The reason is quite simple: foods cooked on high heat without water contain preformed AGEs. The higher the preformed dietary AGE consumption, the greater your oxidative stress and inflammation load.

We understand that avoiding all AGE-containing foods is virtually impossible. We are simply underscoring that a low AGE is one of the most important steps you can take in maintaining your skin younger. Making decisions to boil, steam, and stew will significantly reduce your AGE load. As an example, the decision to boil chicken for a meal as opposed to deciding to oven-fire will reduce your AGE load by ninefold. Poaching an egg instead of frying it in a pan will reduce your AGE load by fivefold. See page 65 for more comparisons, but similar expectations can be made for other water versus oven and skillet choices.

Take a leaf out of the traditional Japanese cooking style—use water, and lots of it, for cooking. Remember that conventional ovens are a recent addition to small Japanese kitchens, and many of the best traditional Japanese meals are prepared for the family in a simmering pot placed on the center of the table.

We said it earlier, and it bears repeating again: a consistently high intake of dietary AGEs is the nutritional equivalent of putting your face in front of a sunlamp. The oxidative stress and inflammation induced by high-AGE foods is an indisputable scientific fact, and we are astonished that it has flown under the radar of nutritionists and other experts working in the beauty field.

Another note worth mentioning is related to fruits and berries. Yes, they do contain important antioxidant chemicals that offer wonderful collagen and UV-protection. Yes, they contain chemicals that help protect the blood vessels that keep the blood flowing smoothly to the skin. However, more and more is not always better. Too much of the fruit sugar fructose is not a good thing for your collagen.

Excess fructose due to a heavy reliance upon dietary fruits as a calorie source is a promoter of AGE destruction in the body. This fact is often overlooked in books and articles by self-proclaimed "nutritionists to the stars" who seem to tout a fruitarian lifestyle with fructose-rich smoothies for breakfast, lunch, and dinner. Ultimately these "star" clients will need extra help from cosmetic dermatologists if they adhere to the fructose plan.

Rather than fill our recipe section with smoothies, puddings, parfaits, and other fruit-containing desserts, we only included three to reflect the need to keep fruit sugars to a moderate level. There is no set rule that determines a line not to cross with regard to fruit sugars; it is simply a judgment call one makes to not overindulge in fruits. Somewhere between our current lack of dietary fruit *variety* and an all-out fruit diet is the middle ground.

Experts from Harvard recommend two to three servings of fruit and an unlimited "abundance" of vegetables daily. The dermatologists of the 1940s were warning against the excesses of fruit sugars, particularly from juice, and we tend to agree with them. Some is good, more is not necessarily better. Alternating between a daily handful of whole grapes, cherries, blueberries, acai, and other deeply colored fruits—particularly the red-purple colors— will protect the skin in moderation.

Making every effort to eliminate pure fructose as an added sugar in other foods and drinks (staying away from high-fructose corn syrup and anything with the word *fructose* in the ingredient list of foods and drinks) will allow room to intake moderate fructose in its true fruit-and-berry context of phytochemical antioxidants and fiber. Whole fruits and berries, with their fibrous skins, are obviously a better choice than bottled juice.

We are grateful to our culinary consultant, Yoshiko Sato of Tokyo, Japan, who helped to infuse a Japanese flavor into some of the low-AGE meals. Let them serve as a reminder that boiling, stewing, steaming, and simmering are options that often tend to be overlooked when researchers talk about the healthy aspects of the traditional Japanese diet. Meals are suitable for two people. Enjoy!

Soups
COLORFUL VEGETABLE CURRY SOUP

3   cups chicken stock
¾   cup zucchini, chopped
¾   cup onion, chopped
⅔   cup eggplant, chopped
⅓   cup orange bell pepper, chopped
1   tablespoon garlic, finely chopped
¾   cup whole tomato, canned or pureed
½   teaspoon curry powder
¼   teaspoon cumin powder
1   tablespoon organic canola oil
       Sea salt, to taste
       Freshly ground black pepper, to taste

Combine the stock, all vegetables, and the chopped garlic in a large pot. Boil for 8 to 10 minutes. Add in the tomato puree, and curry and cumin powders, and stir. Add the canola oil, sea salt, and pepper, and simmer for an additional 5 minutes.

EGGPLANT MISO SOUP

2   cups water
3   tablespoons miso paste
1   cup Japanese eggplant, cut into strips

2 green onions, chopped

¼ teaspoon low-sodium soy sauce

Bring the water to a boil in a medium pot, and add the miso paste, stirring until dissolved. Add the eggplant, and cook 5 minutes. Add the green onions, turn off the heat, and stir in the soy sauce just before serving.

GINGER CHICKEN SOUP WITH SHITAKE

3 cups chicken stock

½ pound chicken breast fillets, cubed to less than 1 inch

⅔ cup carrots, chopped

⅔ cup shiitake mushroom, sliced

½ cup celery, sliced

1 tablespoon ginger, finely chopped

1 tablespoon soy sauce

Sea salt, to taste

Freshly ground black pepper, to taste

Bring the stock to a boil in a medium pot. Add the chicken, carrots, shiitake, celery, and ginger. Slow cook on low heat for 20 minutes. Add the soy sauce, and season with sea salt and pepper.

JAPANESE PUMPKIN-TOFU SOUP

3 cups vegetable stock

¾ pound kabocha pumpkin (or acorn squash), skin and seeds removed, cut into medium cubes

⅔ cup onion, sliced

4 ounces soft or silken tofu, drained

¾ cup rice milk

1 tablespoon canola oil

Sea salt, to taste

Freshly ground black pepper, to taste

1 tablespoon parsley

Bring the vegetable stock to a boil in a large pot. Add the kabocha (or acorn squash) and onion, cooking on medium heat for about 15 to 20 minutes with an occasional stir. Cool and transfer kabocha to a large blender. Add the tofu, and puree until smooth. Return the blended ingredients to the pot on very low heat. Add the rice milk and canola oil, and season with sea salt and black pepper. Ready in just a few minutes. Garnish with parsley.

KIMCHI-MISO SOUP

3⅓   cups chicken stock
⅓   cup shiitake mushrooms, sliced
3   cups bok choy
1   tablespoon garlic, finely chopped
¾   cup kimchi, chopped
2   tablespoons miso paste
1   teaspoon soy sauce
5   ounces firm tofu, cut into 1-inch cubes
½   teaspoon sesame oil
1   tablespoon sesame, ground

Bring the chicken stock to a boil in a medium pot. Add in the shiitake, bok choy, garlic, and kimchi. Cook 5 to 7 minutes. Add in the miso and soy sauce, and stir until well blended. Add in the tofu, and simmer for an additional 2 minutes. Mix in the sesame oil and ground sesame just before serving.

PUMPKIN-MISO SOUP

3   cups water
2   cups kabocha (Japanese pumpkin) or acorn squash
      (cubed, skinned, and pitted)
2   tablespoons miso paste
½   teaspoon of dashi stock or soy sauce
1   tablespoon green onion, chopped

Bring the water to a boil in a medium pot. Add the kabocha, and cook for 7 to 10 minutes until soft. Add the miso paste and dashi stock; stir until well blended. Remove from the heat, and add the green onion prior to serving.

RED PEPPER SOUP

2   cups tomato juice
2   large red bell peppers, chopped

1   small clove garlic

1¾ cups prepared vegetable stock

1   tablespoon olive oil

    Pinch cayenne pepper

    Sea salt, to taste

    Freshly ground black pepper, to taste

    Fresh parsley, chopped

    Nuts

Add the tomato juice, bell peppers, and garlic to a food processor or large blender, and puree. Transfer the mixture to a large cooking pot, and add the stock and the remaining ingredients. Simmer on very low heat for 10 to 15 minutes. Garnish with fresh chopped parsley and nuts of choice. An alternate includes adding ¼ teaspoon of cumin and a pinch of garlic powder.

SALMON AND VEGGIE MISO SOUP

3   cups water

1   cup red or purple potato, chopped

¼   cup asparagus spears, chopped

1   fillet salmon, approximately ¾ pound, cut into quarters

1   tablespoon miso paste

½   teaspoon soy sauce

1   tablespoon green onion, chopped

    Pinch freshly ground black pepper

Bring the water to a boil in a medium pot, and add the potatoes, asparagus, and salmon. Cook for 5 to 7 minutes. Add in the miso paste and soy sauce, stirring until well blended. Remove from heat, and add the green onion and black pepper just prior to serving.

SHRIMP RICE NOODLE SOUP

3¾ cups vegetable stock

1   tablespoon ginger, chopped

2   cups bok choy, chopped

1   cup shiitake mushrooms, sliced

¼   pound rice noodles (pre-soaked in warm water for 1 hour)

8   medium shrimp, shelled and deveined
1   teaspoon sesame oil
     Sea salt, to taste
     Freshly ground black pepper, to taste

Bring the stock to a boil in a large pot. Add the ginger, bok choy, and mushrooms. Simmer for 3 minutes. Add the rice noodles and shrimp, cooking for an additional 3 to 7 minutes. Serve and top with sesame oil. Add sea salt and pepper.

SWEET POTATO CARROT SOUP

3   cups vegetable broth
1   large sweet potato, washed, cut into chunks with
     skin on
2   large carrots, chopped
1   cup onion, chopped
1   tablespoon garlic, chopped
1   tablespoon canola oil
1   teaspoon finely chopped ginger
½   teaspoon garam masala
¼   teaspoon ground turmeric
¼   teaspoon ground cumin powder
     Sea salt, to taste
     Freshly ground black pepper, to taste

Bring the vegetable broth to a boil in a large pot. Add all the ingredients, except the salt and pepper. Cover and simmer on very low heat for 45 minutes to 1 hour. Transfer to a large blender and puree, or use a hand-held blending mechanized stick. Add sea salt and pepper.

TURKEY MEATBALLS IN BOK CHOY SOUP

½   pound ground turkey
1   tablespoon green onion, chopped
1   tablespoon ginger, finely chopped
3   cups chicken stock
2   cups bok choy

Sea salt, to taste

Freshly ground black pepper, to taste

Combine the turkey, green onion, and fresh ginger in a large bowl. Shape the mixture into small meatballs. In a medium pot, bring the chicken stock to a boil, and add the turkey meatballs and bok choy. Simmer for 10 minutes, and add the sea salt and black pepper.

WAKAME TOFU SOUP

2 cups water

5 ounces medium tofu, cubed to 1 inch

1 tablespoon dried wakame seaweed flakes

2 tablespoons miso paste

½ teaspoon dashi stock

Bring the water to a boil in a medium pot. Add the tofu and wakame. Simmer for 3 minutes, and add the miso paste and dashi stock, stirring for at least 1 minute until well blended. Ready to serve.

Salads

ANCHOVY SPINACH SALAD

4 cups romaine lettuce, chopped

2 cups spinach leaves

3 ounces fresh mozzarella, cut into small segments

6 cherry tomatoes, halved

1 can anchovies in olive oil (with or without capers)

Lemon juice, to taste

Freshly ground black pepper, to taste

Combine the lettuce, spinach, mozzarella cheese, and cherry tomatoes in a large salad bowl. Place the anchovies and olive oil on top. Add lemon juice and black pepper.

COLLAGEN-BOOSTING AVOCADO SALAD WITH LIME
Avocado Salad

½ pound medium shrimp, shelled and deveined

8 cherry tomatoes, halved

4   cups romaine lettuce, chopped
1   cup purple onion, thinly sliced and soaked in water
      for 10 minutes
1   cup watercress, chopped
1   medium avocado, skinned, pitted, and sliced
1   medium blood orange, peeled and sliced
1   medium lime, quartered

Vinaigrette Dressing

2   tablespoons extra-virgin olive oil
½   tablespoon Dijon mustard
½   teaspoon rice vinegar
½   teaspoon dried parsley
      Pinch freshly ground black pepper

Boil the shrimp for approximately 3 minutes in a medium pot; remove and cool. Prepare the dressing by combining the ingredients in a small bowl and briefly stirring or whisking. In a large salad bowl, combine the additional vegetables; add the avocado slices, blood orange, and shrimp. Add the dressing and lime to taste.

GREEN TEA SOBA SALAD

3   ounces fresh string beans, tips removed, cut into thirds
¼   pound green-tea soba noodles
1   tablespoon olive oil
5   ounces extra-firm tofu, drained, cubed to 1 inch
8   cherry tomatoes, halved
1   tablespoon black sesame seeds
1   tablespoon organic canola oil
      Sea salt, to taste
      Freshly ground black pepper, to taste

Boil the string beans for 7 to 10 minutes in a medium pot. Remove from the heat, drain, and cool. In a separate pot, boil the green-tea soba for 6 to 7 minutes or to desired firmness. Stir occasionally. Drain the soba, and rinse with cold water; then add the soba to a large salad bowl and mix the olive oil over the noodles. Add the tofu, beans, tomatoes, sesame seeds, and canola oil. Season with sea salt and black pepper. Individually dress with Japanese-style ginger dressing, if desired.

LOWEST AGE CHICKEN WITH CUCUMBER SALAD
Chicken and Cucumber Salad

¾   pound chicken fillet

2   medium tomatoes, sliced

1   large cucumber, cut into thin matchsticks

Ginger Dressing

⅔   cup chopped parsley

¼   cup onion, chopped

1   tablespoon ginger, chopped

3   tablespoons rice vinegar

3   tablespoons organic canola oil

3   tablespoons soy sauce

Combine the ginger dressing ingredients, and puree with a handheld blender or food processor. In a medium pot, bring the water to a boil and add the chicken fillets for 4 to 5 minutes. Drain, cool, and pull the fillets into strips. Place the sliced tomatoes on a plate, and add the cucumber matchsticks on top. Then add the chicken, and finish with Yoshi's ginger dressing.

MOZZARELLA SALAD
Salad

4   cups mixed greens

½   cup watercress, chopped

½   cup purple onion, thinly sliced and soaked in water
     10 minutes

⅔   fresh Italian parsley

3½ ounces fresh mozzarella cheese, sliced

8   black olives

Dressing

3   tablespoons extra-virgin olive oil

1   tablespoon rice vinegar

½   tablespoon fresh lemon juice

Combine the mixed greens, watercress, onion, and parsley in a large salad bowl. Place the fresh mozzarella slices and black olives on top, and add the dressing.

PURPLE POWER SALAD

2   cups purple cauliflower

1   cup purple onion, thinly sliced

½   red apple, cut into thin wedges with skin on

2   tablespoons parsley, medium chopped

Boil the cauliflower in a large pot for about 5 minutes, or less to maintain crispness. Drain and refrigerate. Add the sliced onion and apples to separate bowls of water, and steep for a few minutes. The water for the apple should be lightly salted. Mix all the ingredients together in a large salad bowl. Add your favorite dressing and nuts.

RED AND BLACK BEAN SALAD

⅛   teaspoon ground cumin powder

⅛   teaspoon garam masala

⅛   teaspoon ground turmeric

2   tablespoons organic canola oil

20   ounces canned red and black beans

6   cherry tomatoes, halved

½   cup purple onion, finely chopped

½   cup chopped cilantro

½   cup medium red bell pepper, chopped

2   tablespoons green onion, chopped

2   tablespoons olive oil

1   tablespoon lime juice

3   cups romaine lettuce, chopped

On this rare occasion, we are using pan heat to set up the spices. Heat the cumin, garam masala, and turmeric in 2 tablespoons of canola oil in a pan over medium heat. In a large salad bowl, add the beans, tomatoes, purple onions, cilantro, bell pepper, and green onions. Combine the olive oil with the spices and lime juice, then mix into the salad. Serve on romaine lettuce.

SHABU-SHABU BEEF SALAD
Beef Salad

1 tablespoon ginger, finely chopped
½ pound beef rib-eye, very thinly sliced
8 cherry tomatoes
4 cups dark green lettuce, chopped
½ cup purple onion, thinly sliced and soaked in water
   for 10 minutes
   Freshly squeezed lemon juice, to taste

Sesame Dressing

1 tablespoon sesame oil
1 tablespoon rice vinegar
1 tablespoon soy sauce
1 tablespoon black sesame seeds, ground

Prepare the dressing by combining the ingredients in a small bowl and briefly stirring or whisking. Boil water in a medium pot, and add the chopped ginger and beef. Cook time for shabu-shabu depends on the thickness of the meat. Very thin beef requires much less than one minute of swirling in the hot water before removing. In a large salad bowl, combine the vegetables, and add the cooled beef and dressing. Sprinkle with lemon juice.

TOFU GREEK SALAD
Tofu Salad

4   cups romaine lettuce, chopped
10 cherry tomatoes, halved
1¾ cups cucumber, sliced
1¼ cups purple onion, thinly sliced
¾   cup orange bell peppers, chopped
11 ounces extra-firm tofu, drained and cubed to 1 inch

Pinch sea salt

Freshly ground black pepper, to taste

Dressing

3   tablespoons extra virgin olive oil

1   tablespoon rice vinegar

½   tablespoon fresh lemon juice

½   tablespoon dry oregano

Combine the lettuce, tomatoes, cucumbers, purple onion, and bell pepper in a large salad bowl. Blend together the dressing ingredients in a small bowl. Place the tofu cubes on the top of the salad, and add dressing. Season with sea salt and black pepper.

TOFU SALAD WITH YOSHI'S GINGER DRESSING

Salad Base

4   cups chopped romaine lettuce

4   cups mixed greens with radicchio

5   ounces box extra-firm tofu, drained and cubed to 1 inch

Ginger Dressing

⅔   cup chopped parsley

¼   cup onion, chopped

1   tablespoon ginger, chopped

3   tablespoons rice vinegar

3   tablespoons organic canola oil

3   tablespoons soy sauce

Combine the ginger dressing ingredients, and puree with a handheld blender or food processor. Mix the greens in a large salad bowl, and dress with tofu and ginger dressing.

WHOLE-WHEAT SALMON PASTA SALAD

1⅔ cups organic whole-wheat pasta

1   tablespoon extra virgin olive oil

8   cherry tomatoes, halved

⅔   cup fresh parsley, chopped

½   cup red bell pepper, chopped

½   cup cucumber, finely chopped

¼   cup radish, thinly sliced

3½ ounces wild salmon, canned

1   tablespoon fresh lemon juice

Salt, to taste

Freshly ground black pepper, to taste

Boil pasta in a large pot to desired firmness. Drain, mix in olive oil, and add to a large salad bowl. Add in the tomatoes, parsley, red pepper, cucumber, radish, and salmon. Mix in the fresh lemon, salt, and pepper.

WILD EDAMAME SALAD

8   medium shrimp, deveined

1   cup wild rice

2   tablespoons rice vinegar

1   teaspoon honey

1   teaspoon lemon juice

2   tablespoons olive oil

Sea salt, to taste

Freshly ground black pepper, to taste

1   small carrot, finely chopped

½   orange bell pepper, finely chopped

½   cucumber, finely chopped

½   cup frozen edamame (soy) beans, shells removed

1   tablespoon green onion, chopped

Boil the shrimp for 3 to 4 minutes and set aside. Cook the wild rice in lightly salted water according to the package directions, and let cool. Combine the rice vinegar, honey, lemon juice, olive oil, sea salt, and black pepper. Add the cool wild rice, and then combine the vegetables, shrimp, and finally edamame. Garnish with green onion.

WILD SMOKED SALMON SALAD

8   cherry tomatoes, halved

2   cups baby spinach leaves

2   cups red cabbage, shredded

½   cup purple onion, thinly sliced and soaked in cold
    water for 10 minutes
2   ounces smoked wild salmon in package
2   tablespoons extra-virgin olive oil
½   tablespoon fresh lemon juice
    Sea salt, to taste
    Freshly ground black pepper, to taste

Combine the tomatoes, spinach, red cabbage, and onion in a large salad bowl. Place the wild salmon on top. Add the olive oil and lemon juice, and season with sea salt and black pepper.

Sides
CILANTRO RICE

1   cup brown rice
2   tablespoons canola oil
1   tablespoon garlic, finely chopped
½   cup onion, finely chopped
¼   teaspoon cumin
    Pinch turmeric
1½ tablespoons cilantro, finely chopped

Add the ingredients (except the cilantro) to lightly salted boiling water along with brown rice, per the rice package instructions. (Use a rice maker if desired.) After cooking is completed, softly fold in the cilantro before serving.

STEAMED POWER-VEGGIES

2   cups sweet potato, chopped
2   cups butternut squash, chopped
3   cups broccoli, chopped
2   cups carrots, chopped
2   cups purple cauliflower, chopped
1   cup green beans, halved
    Sea salt, to taste

Add the sweet potato and squash to a large steam pot, and steam for 8 minutes. Add the remainder of the vegetables, and steam all for an additional 5 to 7 minutes. Add the sea salt. This can be served as a stand-alone dish or together with fish or poultry.

STRING BEANS WITH MISO DRESSING

½   pound string beans, tips removed
1   tablespoon miso paste
1   tablespoon fresh ginger juice
1   tablespoon sesame oil
1   tablespoon rice vinegar
1   tablespoon soy sauce
1   tablespoon black sesame seeds, ground

Bring water to a boil in a medium pot. Add the string beans, and cook for 7 to 10 minutes. For miso dressing, combine the additional ingredients in a medium bowl, and mix until well blended. Add the string beans, and mix before serving.

TURMERIC RICE

2   cups vegetable stock
1   cup brown basmati rice
1   tablespoon rice-bran oil
1   teaspoon ground turmeric powder
1   pinch cayenne pepper
1   tablespoon raisins

Bring the vegetable stock to a boil in a pot. Add the rice, oil, turmeric, and cayenne pepper. Cover tightly, and simmer on low heat for about 50 minutes. Remove from heat, and keep covered for 10 minutes. Stir when finished, and add the raisins.

WATERCRESS AND BLACK SESAME

4   cups watercress
1   tablespoon soy sauce
1   teaspoon black sesame seeds, ground
1   tablespoon bonito flakes

Bring water to a boil in a medium pot, and add the watercress for 2 to 3 minutes. Drain and cool, and chop a few times, but not finely. In a medium salad bowl, add the soy sauce, mixing in the ground sesame and watercress. Add the bonito flakes on top before serving.

Smoothies
ACAI-MATCHA PROBIOTIC SMOOTHIE
1   cup rice milk
1   cup soy milk
1   cup frozen blueberries
1   package frozen acai (e.g. Sambazon)
2   tablespoons plain, low-fat yogurt
¼   teaspoon matcha green tea
2   ice cubes

Blend all the ingredients on high and enjoy!

BLACK SESAME PROBIOTIC DELIGHT
12   ounces plain, low-fat yogurt
½   banana, thinly sliced
2   teaspoons black sesame paste or ground black sesame seeds

Mix together and enjoy!

JAPANESE INFUSION PROBIOTIC SMOOTHIE
6   ounces plain, low-fat yogurt
1   cup frozen blueberries
1   teaspoon ground black sesame seeds
½   teaspoon matcha green tea
1½   cups of rice milk (e.g. Rice Dream)
2   ice cubes

Blend all ingredients on high, and enjoy!

Entrées
GINGER-STEAMED WILD SALMON
Salmon and Asparagus
2   wild salmon fillets
2   tablespoons ginger, finely chopped

Sea salt, to taste

Freshly ground black pepper, to taste

10 spears asparagus

Miso Dipping Sauce

1   tablespoon miso paste

1   tablespoon fresh ginger juice

1   tablespoon sesame oil

1   tablespoon rice vinegar

1   tablespoon soy sauce

1   tablespoon black sesame seeds, ground

Add the two fillets of salmon to a large steam pot, and sprinkle on top with the freshly chopped ginger, salt, and black pepper. After 8 minutes of steaming, add the asparagus to the steamer and continue steaming the fish and vegetable for an additional 10 minutes. Prepare the miso dipping sauce by whisking the ingredients together in a small bowl.

LOW-AGE TURKEY AND CABBAGE

1   pound cabbage

¾   pound organic turkey bacon

     Sea salt, to taste

     Freshly ground black pepper, to taste

     Mustard, to taste

Peel the cabbage leaves back, and separate them from the head. Cut each turkey-bacon strip in half. Layer a cabbage leaf and strip of turkey bacon in a steamer pot, alternating between the cabbage and turkey in a sandwich-like fashion. Steam for 8 to 10 minutes on medium heat, adding sea salt and black pepper. Add mustard, if you like, when serving.

MAHI MAHI CURRY

3   cups vegetable stock

2   cups broccoli

¾   cup yellow bell pepper, chopped

¾   carrot, chopped

¾   cup onion, chopped

½   cup mushrooms, sliced

3   tablespoons ground curry powder

1   tablespoon ginger, finely chopped

1   tablespoon garlic, finely chopped

1   bay leaf

1   pound mahi mahi

    Sea salt, to taste

Bring the vegetable stock to a boil in a large pot, and add the broccoli, bell pepper, carrots, onions, mushrooms, ginger, garlic, and bay leaf. Simmer on low heat for 10 minutes. Add the mahi mahi, and cook for an additional 10 minutes on low heat. Finally, add the curry powder and salt. Simmer for an additional 10 minutes. Remove the mahi mahi pieces, and puree or blend the cooled vegetable ingredients with a handheld blender. Add the mahi mahi back to the pot, and serve with brown rice.

SHRIMP AND CABBAGE ROLLS
Shrimp and Cabbage

8   medium shrimp, deveined

4   sheets of 12-inch round rice paper

1   cup red cabbage, shredded

1   small radish, thinly sliced

1   small carrot, shredded

½   cup cilantro, chopped

Ginger Dipping Sauce

⅔   cup chopped parsley

¼   cup onion, chopped

1   tablespoon ginger, chopped

3   tablespoons rice vinegar

3   tablespoons organic canola oil

3   tablespoons soy sauce

Boil the shrimp, and set aside. Add warm-to-hot water (comfortable to hands) to a large, glass cooking bowl. Immerse one rice paper sheet into the water for 10 to 20 seconds, and lay down on a clean, dampened dish towel. Gently wrap all the ingredients (except dipping sauce!) into the rice paper, allowing for a total of 4 rolls. Each roll should be neatly wrapped, approximately 6 inches long and ½ inch wide. Cut if desired. Combine the ginger dipping sauce ingredients, and puree with a hand-held blender or food processor.

WHOLE-WHEAT PASTA AND SARDINE COLLAGEN-PROTECTOR

1⅔ cups organic whole-wheat pasta

2   tablespoons olive oil

8   cherry tomatoes, halved

⅔ cup red bell pepper, chopped

1   can sardines in olive oil and tomato sauce

⅛ teaspoon garlic powder

2   tablespoons parsley, chopped

    Sea salt, to taste

    Freshly ground black pepper, to taste

Boil pasta in a large pot to desired firmness and drain; add 1 tablespoon olive oil and cool. In a large salad bowl, add the pasta, tomatoes, and peppers, mixing with the additional olive oil. Add the sardines; mix lightly, and garnish with garlic powder and chopped parsley. Add sea salt and black pepper.

9

Concluding Remarks

LOOKING BACK ON ALL THE GROUND we have covered in *Your Skin, Younger*, one of the fundamental and rational questions is, "Does it really matter?" In terms of improving the visible signs of aging and delaying their onset through internal nutritional means, the answer is an undeniable yes. We spent a good chunk of our early discussions making the case that a wrinkle is not just a wrinkle. Having an earlier onset of the visible signs of aging is associated with problems in the heart, kidney, and other organ systems.

As we saw in twins studies, the twin who looks older unfortunately risks an earlier death. The twin who lived a difficult life filled with stress, anxiety, and the use of psychiatric drugs had more prominent visible signs of aging. Since nutrition can impact chronic disease states significantly, since the same healthy diet recommended for the prevention of heart disease, diabetes, and neurodegenerative diseases is the same diet that protects against the visible signs of aging and promotes youthful glowing skin, there is no doubt that internal nutrition really matters. There is also no doubt that keeping stress in check really matters. Stress management interventions can help negate inflammatory chemicals and oxidative stress that drive chronic illnesses and visible signs of aging. A good mental outlook, supported by quality nutrition, makes us feel better about ourselves, and that, in turn, promotes a youthful appearance and slows the overall aging process.

But what about topicals and nutritional supplements that address visible signs of aging over the shorter term, such as in thirty to ninety days of use? Do these interventions really matter to our day-to-day quality of life? The research strongly suggests that they do.

Cosmetics and Psychology

There is no doubt that a youthful appearance is associated with higher self-esteem, more confident social interactions, and better overall quality of life. In one study, older adults with fewer visible signs of aging, and who were deemed to be more attractive by third-party assessors, were indeed the ones who reported a more socially outgoing nature and greater life satisfaction. In separate research, independent assessors deemed more attractive older adults to be happier, to have more desirable personality characteristics, and to have excelled in professional ventures.

Cosmetics also have a place in the aging process. A small number of studies have confirmed what most people would presume to be common sense: the use of topical cosmetics has a favorable influence on well-being. Feeling better about oneself, in turn, has a pay-it-forward benefit because it will likely have a positive influence on subsequent social interactions. Indeed, some studies have shown that use of cosmetics alters the perceptions of third-party individuals in a favorable way.

Cosmetic changes can influence third-party ratings of happiness, intelligence, mental adjustment, and perceptions of leadership abilities. Perhaps most telling is a study by psychology professor Judith Waters, PhD. She used photographs of before and after cosmetic makeovers attached to resumes and submitted them to 120 major corporations or recruiters. Based on the same resume, the one submitted with the cosmetic makeover resulted in a salary offer of up to 20 percent higher.

Whether we like it or not, attractiveness ratings as we age are frequently and strongly associated with the visible signs of aging. There is no way to sugar-coat this undeniable fact. The silver lining here is that improving the visible signs of aging through nonsurgical means can have a favorable impact on mental outlook and social confidence. In other words, we don't have to sit idly by and let the facial aging process drag us down.

Two separate studies, both in the *Journal of the American Academy of Dermatology* (1991, 1994), have shown that topical vitamin A (as retinoic acid) can improve visible signs of aging—no surprise there—while also decreasing anxiety and improving comfort levels in social interactions, as opposed to a placebo cream that simply made the skin feel more smooth. These studies teach us that improving the visible signs of aging can indeed improve mental outlook, and since we covered two chapters worth of internal supplements and topical preparations that can improve the visible signs of aging, the expectations there should be no different.

Indeed, the expectations with our internal and external programs of nutrients should arguably be even higher than those for cosmetic topical creams alone when it comes to improving mental outlook. We say this not only because some of our recommended supplements have been shown to improve the visible signs of aging and promote healthy, glowing skin (for example, omega-3 fatty acids, zinc, selenium, and green tea), but also because they have been independently associated with improved mood states. Recall the growing body of research showing that omega-3 fatty acids, especially the skin-friendly EPA, can improve depressive symptoms.

With research in place showing that both internal supplements and external natural, topical preparations improve the visible signs of aging, users can play an active role in maintaining youthful skin. The importance of this cannot be over-estimated because it provides a sense of legitimate control over an inevitable process. Research shows that when older adults lose a sense of personal control over aspects of health, that only contributes to a downward cycle. Once an individual waves the white flag of surrender to aspects of appearance and physical fitness, as is the hallmark of depression, the road to physical ill-health is firmly paved.

Again, this is not to say that supplements and natural, topical skin foods represent a fountain of youth. They don't, nor do stress management, social involvement, physical fitness, eating fish or whole grains, or any combination of these. We are simply making the case that such practices will place you among the individuals who have insulation against the skin-aging process, which will in turn promote an increased likelihood of greater self-esteem and enhanced quality of life. We began our book by making the case that a wrinkle is not just a wrinkle, and we will conclude having made the case that the interventions outlined in our book really do make a difference on many levels.

Collateral Benefits: Not Just a Camouflage

In a cover story on the cosmetics industry more than fifty years ago, *Time* magazine (June 15, 1958) made a prediction that has proven true: "Whatever form the race for beauty and health takes, its tempo is sure to speed up. As medical science enables more people to live longer—and feel younger, they will also want to look younger. Enormous demand will have to be met for special cosmetics for the aged..."

Today, however, we are not simply seeking cosmetics for the aged. We are also seeking preventive lifestyle and nutrient interventions for adults younger than thirty who already see themselves on the road to aging skin. Given the startling study in the *British Journal of Dermatology* (2001) showing that more than half of healthy women *under* the age of thirty are dissatisfied with the appearance of their skin, the timeliness of the scientific advances in nutritional skin care couldn't be better.

Many of the complaints of these young adults, none of whom had eating disorders or mental-health problems, were associated with what might be observed through the aging process—dark circles, hyperpigmentation, and fine lines. This may be dismissed as yet another example of a youth-obsessed culture, and since beauty and success are equated with youth, those on track to middle age may be especially fearful of any sign that visible aging is imminent. However, the heightened awareness of the skin-aging process among younger adults represents an opportunity to educate on lifestyle habits that would otherwise not be adopted. The diet and lifestyle habits advocated in *Your Skin, Younger* have an abundance of collateral health benefits well beyond the appearance of the skin.

Looking Forward and Back

Enormous strides in cosmetic dermatology have allowed clinicians to make in-office changes to visible signs of aging that would not have been fathomed just a few decades ago. Advances in light therapy, injectables, and prescription creams have been reported to improve how patients feel about themselves, and this, in turn, improves quality of life and social interactions.

Yet for us, this is not the time to sit back and assume we can't make a good thing better. The lifestyle changes, the supplements and topical skin foods, the cooking techniques and stress management considerations we advocate are all individually and collectively supportive of the mainstream care provided by the best cosmetic dermatologists. In other words, true holistic care in the promotion of skin health should be fully inclusive of the considerations once held to be of great importance by the dermatology elders.

Too often in the Western world, there is a bias against research that is old. The prevailing attitude of "What did they know?" is really an extension of the ageism we see in society at large. Of course, they didn't know everything, yet in truth they knew plenty. There was a great wisdom that is only now starting to become fully appreciated. Alternatively, some "new" discoveries are not new at all. We have known about much of the fundamental content of this book for almost a century, yet it would sound more exciting if we claimed to have discovered something.

The only thing we can claim in this book is to have made a strong argument for change—change in the way we view facial aging as benign, change in the atrocious dietary habits we have, change in the way we burden ourselves with stressors, and change in the way we view the gastrointestinal tract as it relates to the skin and brain.

To make our argument, we have woven together thousands of published studies, many of them with the ink hardly dry, and countless others deeply rooted in history. We hope that our small contributions will bring credit to the dermatologists and scientists who deserve it. We didn't make the pH-diet and skin connection; that was done one hundred years ago. We aren't the first to advocate for lots of fish and seafood for the prevention of wrinkles; Manhattan dermatologist Irwin Lubowe did so more than twenty-five years ago. We didn't discover the connection between friendly intestinal bacteria and skin health; others did decades ago.

All three of your authors will continue to research and strive for advances based on forward-thinking, cutting-edge research. We will also continue to look back into the rich history of dermatology, assured that more treasures are waiting to be identified in the "dustbin of history." We will continue in our efforts, turning over all the stones possible in our attempt to promote youthful, glowing skin and its ultimate goal—overall wellness.

For your part, remember that the dietary decisions you make are not without consequence to your collagen, and stress unmanaged is a wrinkle in the making. Many aspects of the long-term care of your skin require your active participation, all the while maintaining your skin, younger!

Alan C. Logan, ND   Mark G. Rubin, MD   Phillip M. Levy, MD

Appendices

Resources

More on Alan C. Logan, ND

http://www.drlogan.com

Nutritionally Oriented Medical Doctors and Naturopathic Physicians

American Holistic Medical Association
23366 Commerce Park, Suite 101B
Beachwood, OH 44122
Phone: 216-292-6644
FAX: 216-292-6688
http://www.holisticmedicine.org

American Association of Naturopathic Physicians
4435 Wisconsin Ave. NW, Suite 403
Washington, DC 20016
Phone: 202-237-8150
FAX: 202-237-8152
Toll free: 1-866-538-2267
http://www.naturopathic.org

Canadian Association of Naturopathic Doctors
26 Holly St., Suite 200
Toronto, Ontario, Canada M4S 3B1
Phone: 416-496-8633
FAX: 416-496-8634
Toll free: 1-800-551-4381
http://www.cand.ca

Mind-Body Medicine Programs and Resources

Benson-Henry Institute for Mind-Body Medicine
151 Merrimac St.
Boston, MA 02114
Phone: 617-643-6090
FAX: 617-643-6077
Contact: mindbody@partners.org
http://www.mbmi.org

The Center for Mind-Body Medicine
5225 Connecticut Ave. NW, Suite 414
Washington, DC 20015
Phone: 202-966-7338
http://www.cmbm.org

Environmental, Chemical Contaminants in Food and Cosmetics

The Environmental Working Group
1436 U St. NW, Suite 100
Washington, DC 20009
Phone: 202-667-6982
http://www.ewg.org
Provides up-to-date information on:
    1. Safety of cosmetic ingredients. (See the "Skin Deep" area of the site.)
    2. Mercury and toxins in fish and seafood.
    3. Pesticides on North American produce.

Omega-3 Supplement Independent Quality Assurance
International Fish Oil Standards
120 Research Lane, Suite 203
University of Guelph Research Park
Guelph, Ontario, Canada N1G 0B4
Toll free: 877-557-7722
http://www.ifosprogram.com
Provides public disclosure of independent testing on commercial fish-oil supplements.

Nutritional Supplements for Skin
Genuine Health Inc.
317 Adelaide St. West, Suite 501
Toronto, Ontario, Canada M5V 1P9
Phone: 416-977-3505
Toll free: 877-500-7888
http://www.genuinehealth.com
Genuine Health is a science-based company that provides high-quality, safe, and effective natural products. They work closely with scientists and have conducted original research on products at the University of Toronto and other prestigious institutions.

Genuine Health's Healthy Skin Program—Genuine Beauty— includes a number of high-quality oral supplements and topical deodorized fish oil for the promotion of healthy, youthful skin.

Kyolic Aged Garlic
Wakunaga of America Co., Ltd.
23501 Madero
Mission Viejo, CA 92691 USA
1-800-421-2998
www.kyolic.com

Super Glisodin
Novus Research, Inc.
#223, 745 North Gilbert Road, Ste 124
Gilbert, Arizona 85234
1-800-244-2438
www.superglisodin.com

Natural Cosmetics: Premium Body Care Standards
Whole Foods Market, Inc.
550 Bowie St.
Austin, TX 78703
Phone: 512-477-4455
Voicemail: 512-477-5566
FAX: 512-482-7000
http://www.wholefoodsmarket.com
To find the section on Premium Body Care Standards, look under the
"Health and Nutrition" heading on the website home page.

Sleep Beverage
zenbev
Biosential Inc.
1543 Bayview Ave., Suite 346
Toronto, Ontario, Canada M4G 3B5
Phone: 416-421-7445
Toll free: 800-735-4538
http://www.zenbev.com

Probiotics
Bifidobacterium infantis 35624 (Align)***
Procter & Gamble
1 Procter & Gamble Plaza
Cincinnati, OH 45202
Toll-free: 1-800-208-0112
http://www.aligngi.com

***This highly researched probiotic is proven to lower inflammatory markers outside the gut.

Lactobacillus plantarum 299V (LactoFlamX)
Metagenics, Inc.
9770 44th Ave. NW, Suite 100
Gig Harbor, WA 98332
Toll free: 1-800-843-9660
http://www.metagenics.com

Lactobacillus casei Strain Shirota (Yakult)
Yakult U.S.A. Inc.
3625 Del Amo Blvd., Suite 260
Torrance, CA 90503
Phone: 310-542-7065
FAX : 310-542-7045
http://www.yakultusa.com

Lactobacillus GG (Culturelle)
Amerifit Brands
55 Sebethe Drive, Suite 102
Cromwell, CT 06416
Toll free: 1-800-722-3476
http://www.culturelle.com

Natren Inc. Probiotics
3105 Willow Ln.
Westlake Village, CA 91361
1-866-462-8736
www.natren.com

Rachel's Dairy
12002 Airport Way
Broomfield, CO 80021
1-888-841-1112
www.rachelsdairy.com

Stonyfield Farm
10 Burton Drive
Londonderry, NH 03053
1-800-776-2697
www.stonyfield.com

Biofeedback Supplies for Meditation and Mind-Body Exercises

Biodot of Indiana, Inc.
P.O. Box 1207
Bedford, IN 47421
Toll free: 1-800-272-2340
http://www.biodots.net

StressEraser
Helicor, Inc.
25 Washington St., Suite 526
Brooklyn, NY 11201
Toll free: 888-437-0700
http://www.stresseraser.com

Negative Air Ion Generator

SphereOne, Inc.
945 Main St./P.O. Box 1013
Silver Plume, CO 80476
Phone: 303-569-3236
http://www.sphereone.com

Japanese Foods
Mitsuwa Marketplace
595 River Road
Edgewater, NJ 07020
Phone: 201-941-9113
http://www.mitsuwa.com/english
Also has retail markets in Chicago and six California locations.

Kenko Nutrition
www.kenkonutrition.com
Online source of Japanese Matcha, quality teas, green tea noodles, sesame and polyphenol-rich chocolate.

Nutrition Information and Traditional Regional Diets
Oldways Preservation & Exchange Trust
266 Beacon St.
Boston, MA 02116
Phone: 617-421-5500
FAX: 617-421-5511
http://www.oldwayspt.org
Oldways is a widely respected not-for-profit, food-issues think tank praised for translating the complex details of nutrition science into "the familiar language of food." This synthesis converts high-level science into a consumer-friendly health-promotion tool. Jointly with the Harvard School of Public Health and other institutions, Oldways has published the "healthy eating pyramids," a set of guides based on worldwide dietary traditions closely associated with good health.

References

Introduction and Chapter 1: Inside Out: The Renewed Science of Dermatology

Adams, et al. "Status of nutrition education in medical schools." *Am J Clin Nutr* 2006;83(4):941S–944S.

Borkan, et al. "Comparison of visually estimated age with physiologically predicted age as indicators of rates of aging." *Soc Sci Med* 1982;16:197–204.

Burr and Burr. "A new deficiency disease produced by the rigid exclusion of fat from the diet." *J Biol Chem* 1929;82:345–367.

Choi, Maibach. "Role of ceramides in barrier function of healthy and diseased skin." *Am J Clin Dermatol* 2005;6:215–223.

Christensen, et al. "Looking old for your age: genetics and mortality." *Epidemiology* 2004;15:251–252.

Cordain, et al. "Origins and evolution of the Western diet: health implications for the 21st century." *Am J Clin Nutr* 2005;81(2):341–354.

Cosgrove, et al. "Dietary nutrient intakes and skin-aging appearance among middle-aged American women." *Am J Clin Nutr* 2007;86:1225–1231.

Craig and Beck. "Phytochemicals: health protective effects." *Can J Diet Pract Res* 1999 Summer;60(2):78–84.

Daniell. "Smoker's wrinkles: a study in the epidemiology of 'crow's feet.'" *Ann Intern Med* 1971 Dec;75(6):873–880.

Denomme, et al. "Directly quantitated dietary (n–3) fatty acid intakes of pregnant Canadian women are lower than current dietary recommendations." *J Nutr* 2005;135(2):206–311.

Dattner. "The IVth IACD Congress—a holistic perspective." *J Cosmet Dermatol* 2006;5:178–80.

Dattner. "Nutritional dermatology." *Clin Dermatol* 1999;17:57–64.

Fore. "A review of skin and the effects of aging on skin structure and function." *Ostomy Wound Management* 2006;52:24–35.

Grove. "Age-related differences in the healing of superficial skin wounds in humans." *Arch Dermatol Res* 1982;272:381–385.

Guenther, et al. "Most Americans eat much less than recommended amounts of fruits and vegetables." *J Am Diet Assoc* 2006;106(9):1371–1379.

Guyuron, et al. "Factors contributing to the facial aging of identical twins." *Plast Reconstruct Surg* 2009;123:1321–1331.

Kant, et al. "Reported consumption of low-nutrient-density foods by American children and adolescents: nutritional and health correlates, NHANES III, 1988 to 1994." *Arch Pediatr Adolesc Med* 2003;157(8):789–796.

Kilgman and Dattner. "Toward optimal health: the experts respond to aging skin." *J Womens Health Gend Based Med* 1999 Oct;8(8):1021–5.

Mariman. "Nutrigenomics and nutrigenetics: the 'omics' revolution in nutritional science." *Biotechnol Appl Biochem* 2006 Jun;44(Part 3): 119–128.

Nanney, et al. "Examination of the adherence to the '5 A Day the Color Way' campaign among parents and their preschool children." *J Cancer Edu* 2007;22:177–180.

Park, et al. "Facial wrinkles as a predictor of decreased renal function." *Nephrology* 2008;13:522–527.

Purba, et al. "Can skin wrinkling in a site that has received limited sun exposure be used as a marker of health status and biological age?" *Age Ageing* 2001 May;30(3):227–234.

Purba, et al. "Skin wrinkling: can food make a difference?" *J Am Coll Nutr* 2001 Feb;20(1):71–80.

Rexbye, et al. "Influence of environmental factors on facial ageing." *Age Ageing* 2006 Mar;35(2):110–115.

Schnor, et al. "Gray hair, baldness, and wrinkles in relation to myocardial infarction: the Copenhagen City Heart Study." *Am Heart J* 1995;130: 1003–1010.

Scott-Kantor. "Many Americans are not meeting food guide pyramid dietary recommendations." *Food Review* 1996;18:7–15.

Shepherd and Linn. "Evaluation of vitamin F." *Drug Cosmet Industry* 1936;38:629.

Simopoulos, et al. "Workshop on the essentiality of and recommended dietary intakes for omega-6 and omega-3 fatty acids." *J Am Coll Nutr* 1999 Oct;18(5):487–489.

Sinclair. "Essential fatty acids—an historical perspective." *Biochem Soc Trans* 1990;18:756–761.

Sinclair. "Nutrition and the skin in man." *Ann Nutr Aliment* 1957;11: A147–176.

Spencer, et al. "Predictors of nutrition counseling behaviors and attitudes in U.S. medical students." *Am J Clin Nutr* 2006 Sep;84(3):655–662.

Stokes, et al. *Fundamentals of Medical Dermatology.* University of Pennsylvania, Department of Dermatology Book Fund, 1942.

White. "The elastic tissue of the skin." *J Cutaneous Dis* 1910;4:163–247.

Chapter 2: Inflammation and Oxidative Stress: The Flames of Skin Aging

Ayata, et al. "Oxidative stress–mediated skin damage in an experimental mobile phone model can be prevented by melatonin." *J Dermatol* 2004;31:878–883.

Behrman, et al. "Dermatologic therapy with cod-liver oil ointment." *Ind Med Surg* 1949;18:512–518.

Bendiner. "Disastrous trade-off: Eskimo health for white civilization." *Hosp Pract* 1974;9:156–189.

Berwick. "Counterpoint: sunscreen use is a safe and effective approach to skin cancer prevention." *Cancer Epidemiol Biomarkers Prev* 2007;16:1923–1924.

Black. "Mechanisms of pro- and antioxidation." *J Nutr* 2004;134:3169S–3170S.

Black and Rhodes. "The potential of omega-3 fatty acids in the prevention of non-melanoma skin cancer." *Cancer Detection Prev* 2006;30: 224–232.

Bralley, et al. "Inhibition of hyaluronidase activity by select sorghum brans." *J Med Food* 2008;11:307–312.

Brosche and Platt. "Effect of borage-oil consumption on fatty acid metabolism, transepidermal water loss, and skin parameters in elderly people." *Arch Gerontol Geriatr* 2000;30:139–150.

Brown, et al. "Effect of vitamin E deficiency on collagen metabolism in the rat's skin." *J Nutr* 1967;91(1):99–106.

Brusch, Johnson. "A new dietary regimen for arthritis." *J Nat Med Assoc* 1959;51:266–270.

Burke. "Interaction of vitamins C and E as better cosmeceuticals." *Dermatologic Ther* 2007;20:314–321.

Butterworth. "The role of heredity in acne vulgaris." *Penn Med J* 1941;44:1162–1165.

Cho, et al. "Anti-wrinkling effects of the mixture of vitamin C, vitamin E, pycnogenol and evening primrose oil, and molecular mechanisms on hairless mouse skin caused by chronic ultraviolet B irradiation." *Photodermatol Photoimmunol Photomed* 2007;23:155–162.

Cimino, et al. "Protective effects of a red orange extract on UVB-induced damage in human keratinocytes." *Biofactors* 2007;30:129–138.

Clough-Gorr, et al. "Exposure to sunlamps, tanning beds, and melanoma risk." *Cancer Causes Control* 2008;19:659–669.

Cluver. "Sun trauma prevention." *S Africa Med J* 1964;38:801–803.

Darvin, et al. "Cutaneous concentration of lycopene correlates significantly with the roughness of the skin." *Eur J Pharm Biopharm* 2008;69:943–947.

Darvin, et al. "One-year study on the variation of carotenoid antioxidant substances in living human skin: influence of dietary supplementation and stress factors." *J Biomed Optics* 2008;13:044028.

De Spirt, et al. "Intervention with flaxseed and borage-oil supplements modulates skin condition in women." *Br J Nutr* 2008;101:440–445.

Eberlein-Konig, et al. "Protective effect against sunburn of combined systemic ascorbic acid and d–α–tocopherol." *J Am Acad Dermatol* 1998;38:45–48.

Esposito and Giugliano. "Whole-grain intake cools down inflammation." *Am J Clin Nutr* 2006;83(6):1440–1441.

Fisher, et al. "Collagen fragmentation promotes oxidative stress and elevates matrix metalloproteinase-1 in fibroblasts in aged human skin." *Am J Path* 2009;174:101–114.

Fuchs and Kern. "Modulation of UV-light-induced skin inflammation by d–α–tocopherol and L-ascorbic acid: a clinical study using solar simulated radiation." *Free Rad Biol Med* 1998;25:1006–1012.

Garland, et al. "Could sunscreens increase melanoma risk?" *Am J Pub Health* 1992;82:614–615.

Giacomoni, Rein. "Factors of skin aging share common mechanisms." *Biogerontology* 2001;2:219–229.

Gitto, et al. "Individual and synergistic antioxidant actions of melatonin: studies with vitamin E, vitamin C, glutathione, and desferioxamine in rat liver homogenates." *J Pharm Pharmacol* 2001; 53:1393–1401.

Glavind, Christensen. "Influence of nutrition and light on the peroxide content of the skin surface lipids of rats." *Acta Derm-Venereol* 1967;47:339–344.

Godaqr, et al. "UV doses of young adults." *Photochem Photobiol* 2003;77:453–457.

Hallberg. "A reduced repair efficiency can explain increasing melanoma rates." *Eur J Cancer Prev* 2008;17:147–152.

Hanson, et al. "Sunscreen enhancement of UV-induced reactive oxygen species in the skin." *Free Radic Med* 2006;41:1205–1212.

Hardell, et al. "Cellular and cordless telephones and basal cell carcinoma." *Arch Environ Health* 2003;58:380–382.

Heikkinen, et al. "Effects of mobile phone radiation on UV-induced skin tumorigenesis in ornithine decarboxylase transgenic and non-transgenic mice." *Int J Radiat Biol* 2003;79:221–233.

Heinrich, et al. "Antioxidant supplements improve parameters related to skin structure in humans." *Skin Pharm Physiol* 2006;19:224–231.

Heinrich, et al. "Long-term ingestion of high-flavanol cocoa provides photoprotection against UV-induced erythema and improves skin condition in women." *J Nutr* 2006;136(6):1565–1569.

Henderson, et al. "Influence of omega-3 and omega-6 fatty acid sources on prostaglandin levels in mice." *Lipids* 1989;24:502–505.

Horrobin. "Essential fatty acids in clinical dermatology." *J Am Acad Dermatol* 1989;20:1045–1053.

Hwang, et al. "Soy and alfalfa phytoestrogen extracts become potent low-density liporotein antioxidants in the presence of Acerola cherry extract." *J Agric Food Sci* 2001;49:308–314.

Hwang, et al. "Synergistic inhibition of LDL oxidation by phytoestrogens and ascorbic acid." *Free Radic Biol Med* 2000;29:79–89.

Ishihara, et al. "Statistical profiles of malignant melanoma and other skin cancers in Japan: 2007 update." *Int J Clin Oncol* 2008;13:33–41.

Izumi, et al. "Oral intake of soy isoflavone aglycone improves the aged skin of adult women." *J Nutr Sci Vitaminol* 2007;53:57–62.

Kanungo and Patnaik. "Ascorbic acid and aging in the rat." *Biochem J* 1964;90:637–640.

Karinen, et al. "Mobile phone radiation might alter protein expression in human skin." *BMC Genomics* 2008;9:77.

Kim, et al. "6-gingerol prevents UVB-induced ROS production and COX-2 expression *in vitro* and *in vivo*." *Free Rad Res* 2007;41:603–614.

Kromann, et al. "Skin cancer in Greenland 1955–1974." *J Cancer Res Clin Oncol* 1983;105(1):76–78.

Lantz, et al. "The effect of extracts from the ginger rhizome on inflammatory mediator production." *Phytomedicine* 2007;14:123–128.

Lantz, et al. "The effect of turmeric extracts on inflammatory mediator production." *Phytomedicine* 2005;12:445–452.

Lubowe. "A modern approach to the treatment of the aging skin." *J Appl Nutr* 1979;31:64–66.

McCarthy, et al. "Beach holiday sunburn: the sunscreen paradox and gender differences." *Cutis* 1999;64:37–42.

Muggli. "Systemic evening primrose oil improves the biophysical skin parameters of healthy adults." *Int J Cosmet Sci* 2005;27:243–249.

Neukman, et al. "Consumption of flavanol-rich cocoa acutely increases microcirculation in human skin." *Eur J Nutr* 2007;46:53–6.i.

Nole and Johnson. "An analysis of cumulative lifetime solar ultraviolet radiation exposure and the benefits of daily sun protection." *Dermatol Ther* 2004;17:57–62.

Orengo, et al. "Influence of dietary menhaden oil upon carcinogenesis and various cutaneous responses to ultraviolet radiation." *Photochem Photobiol* 1989;49:71–77.

Orengo, et al. "Influence of fish-oil supplementation on the minimal erythema dose in humans." *Arch Dermatol Res* 1992;284:219–21.

Owens, et al. "Influence of wind on chronic ultraviolet light-induced carcinogenesis." *Br J Dermatol* 1977;97:285–287.

Ozguner, et al. "Prevention of mobile phone–induced skin tissue changes by melatonin in rat: an experimental study." *Toxicol Indust Health* 2004;20:133–139.

Palombo, et al. "Beneficial long-term effects of combined oral/topical antioxidant treatment with the carotenoids lutein and zeaxanthin on human skin." *Skin Pharm Physiol* 2007;20:199–210.

Pereda, et al. "Effect of green *Coffea arabica* L. seed oil on extracellular matrix components and water-channel expression in *in vitro* and *ex vivo* human skin models." *J Cosmet Dermatol* 2009;8:56–62.

Pierard. "Ageing in the sun parlour." *Int J Cosmet Sci* 1998;20:251–259.

Pinckney. "The biological toxicity of polyunsaturated fats." *Med Counterpoint* 1973;5:53–71.

Prior and Wu. "Anthocyanins: structural characteristics that result in unique metabolic patterns and biological activities." *Free Radic Res* 2006;40(10):1014–1028.

Puch, et al. "Consumption of functional fermented milk containing borage oil, green tea, and vitamin E enhances skin barrier function." *Exp Dermatol* 2008;17(8):668–674.

Rattner, Sutton. "The aging skin." *Med Clin North Amer* 1956;Jan:33–49.

Rice. "Forty years of omega-3." *Prostaglandins Leukot Essent Fatty Acids* 2008;79:79–81.

Schaffer. "Essential fatty acids and eicosanoids in cutaneous inflammation." *Int J Dermatol* 1989 Jun;28(5):281–290.

Segger, et al. "Supplementation with Eskimo Skin Care improves skin elasticity in women." *J Dermatol Treat* 2008;19:279–283.

Seo, et al. "Enhanced expression of cyclooxygenase-2 by UV in aged human skin *in vivo*." *Mech Ageing Devel* 2003;124:903–910.

Stahl and Sies. "Carotenoids and flavonoids contribute to nutritional protection against skin damage from sunlight." *Mol Biotechnol* 2007;37:26–30.

Stahl, et al. "Carotenoids and carotenoids plus vitamin E protect against ultraviolet light-induced erythema in humans." *Am J Clin Nutr* 2000;71:795–798.

Stahl, et al. "Lycopene-rich products and dietary photoprotection." *Photochem Photobiol Sci* 2006;5:238–242.

Stokes. "Treating the common skin diseases." *GP* 1950;11:33–36.

Straumfjord. "Vitamin A: its effect on acne." *Northwest Med* 1943;42: 219–225.

Tatai, et al. "Effects of vitamin C intake on skin color changes caused by ultraviolet rays." *Chiryo* 1964;46:1315–1318.

Thangapazham, et al. "Beneficial role of curcumin in skin diseases." *Adv Exp Med Biol* 2007;595:343–357.

Thiele, et al. "*In vivo* exposure to ozone depletes vitamins C and E and induces lipid peroxidation in epidermal layers of murine skin." *Free Rad Biol Med* 1997;23:385–391.

Thronfeldt. "Chronic inflammation is etiology of extrinsic aging." *J Cos Dermatol* 2008;7:78–82.

Tsukahara, et al. "Inhibition of ultraviolet B–induced wrinkle formation by an elastase-inhibiting herbal extract: implication for the mechanism underlying elastase-associated wrinkles." *Int J Derm* 2006;45:460–468.

Wu, et al. "Lipophilic and hydrophilic antioxidant capacities of common foods in the United States." *J Agric Food Chem* 2004 Jun 16;52(12):4026–4037.

Yamada, et al. "Dietary tocotrienol reduces UVB-induced skin damage and sesamin enhances tocotrienol effects in hairless mice." *J Nutr Sci Vitaminol* 2008;54:117–123.

Yusuf, et al. "Photoprotective effects of green tea polyphenols." *Photodermatol Photoimmunol Photomed* 2007;23:48–56.

Chapter 3: Sugar and the AGEing Skin

Ahmad, et al. "Aged garlic extract and S-allyl cysteine prevent formation of advanced glycation end-products." *Eur J Pharm* 2007;561:32–38.

Alhamdani, et al. "Decreased formation of advanced glycation end-products in peritoneal fluid by carnosine and related peptides." *Peritoneal Dialysis Int* 2007;27:86–89.

Avery and Bailey. "The effects of the Maillard reaction on the physical properties and cell interactions of collagen." *Pathologie Biologie* 2006;54:387–395.

Babu, et al. "Effect of green tea extract on advanced glycation and cross-linking of tail tendon collagen in streptozotocin-induced diabetic rats." *Food Chem Toxicol* 2008;46:280–285.

Beisswenger, et al. "Ketosis leads to increased methylglycoxal production on the Atkins diet." *Ann NY Acad Sci* 2005;1043:201–210.

Bengmark. "Advanced glycation and lipidoxidation end products—amplifiers of inflammation: the role of food." *J Parenter Enteral Ther* 2007;31:430–440.

Berge, et al. "Sugar-induced premature aging and altered differentiation in human epidermal keratinocytes." *Ann NY Acad Sci* 2007;1100:524–529.

Bray. "Fructose: should we worry?" *Int J Obes* 2008;32:S127–S131.

Cai, et al. "Oral glycotoxins determine the effects of calorie restriction on oxidant stress, age-related diseases, and lifespan." *Am J Path* 2008;173:327–336.

Corstjens, et al. "Glycation-associated skin autofluorescence and skin elasticity are related to chronological age and body mass index of healthy subjects." *Exp Gerontol* 2008;43:663–667.

Dearlove, et al. "Inhibition of protein glycation by extracts of culinary herbs and spices." *J Med Food* 2008;11:275–281.

Delgado-Andrade, et al. "Maillard reaction indicators in diets usually consumed by adolescent population." *Mol Nutr Food Res* 2007;51:341–351.

Duffey and Popkin. "High-fructose corn syrup: is this what's for dinner?" *Am J Clin Nutr* 2008;88:1722S–1732S.

Furber. "Extracellular glycation crosslinks: prospects for removal." *Rejuv Res* 2006;9:274–278.

Gaby. "Adverse effects of dietary fructose." *Altern Med Rev* 2005;10:294–306.

Goldberg, et al. "Advanced glycoxidation end-products in commonly consumed foods." *J Am Diet Assoc* 2004;104:1287–1291.

Hipkiss. "Would carnosine or a carnivorous diet help suppress aging and associated pathologies?" *Ann NY Acad Sci* 2006;1067:369–374.

Jeanmaire, et al. "Glycation during human dermal intrinsic and actinic ageing: an *in vivo* and *in vitro* model." *Br J Dermatol* 2001;145:10–18.

Kallio, et al. "Inflammation markers are modulated by responses to diets differing in postprandial insulin responses in individuals with the metabolic syndrome." *Am J Clin Nutr* 2008;87:1497–1503.

Koschinsky, et al. "Orally absorbed reactive glycation products (glycotoxins): an environmental risk factor in diabetic nephropathy." *Proc Natl Acad Sci* 1997;94:6474–6479.

Krajcovicova-Kudlackova, et al. "Advanced glycation end-products and nutrition." *Physiol Res* 2002;51:313–316.

Levi and Werman. "Long-term fructose consumption accelerates glycation and several age-related variables in male rats." *J Nutr* 1998;128:1442–1449.

Lyons, et al. "Decrease in skin collagen glycation and improved glycemic control in patients with insulin-dependent diabetes." *J Clin Invest* 1991;87:1910–1915.

Masaki, et al. "Generation of active oxygen species from advanced glycation end-products (AGE) under ultraviolet light A irradiation." *Biochem Biophys Res Comm* 1997;235:306–310.

Mikulikova, et al. "Advanced glycation end-product pentosidine accumulates in various tissues of rats with higher fructose intake." *Physiol Res* 2008;57:89–94.

Mills, et al. "Dietary glycated protein modulates the colonic microbiota towards a more detrimental composition in ulcerative colitis patients and non-ulcerative colitis subjects." *J Appl Microbiol* 2008;105:706–714.

Monnier, et al. "Skin collagen-linked fluorescence predicts atherosclerosis progression in the epidemiology of diabetes interventions and complications study." *Ann NY Acd Sci* 2005;1043:917.

Mulder, et al. "Skin autofluorescence, a novel marker for glycemic and oxidative stress-derived advanced glycation end-products." *Diabetes Technol Ther* 2006;8:523–535.

Nandhini, et al. "Taurine prevents fructose-diet induced collagen abnormalities in rat skin." *J Diabetes Compl* 2005;19:305–311.

O'Brien and Morrissey. "Nutrition and toxicological aspects of the Maillard browning reaction in foods." *Crit Rev Food Sci Nutr* 1989;28:211–248.

Odetti, et al. "Age-related increase of collagen fluorescence in human subcutaneous tissue." *Metabolism* 1992;41:655–658.

Pageon, et al. "Reconstructed skin modified by glycation of the dermal equivalent as a model for skin aging and its potential use to evaluate anti-glycation molecules." *Exp Gerontol* 2008;43:584–588.

Peng, et al. "Cinnamon bark proanthocyanidins as reactive carbonyl scavengers to prevent the formation of advanced glycation end-products." *J Agr Food Chem* 2008;56:1907–1911.

Peppa, et al. "Aging and glycoxidant stress." *Hormones* 2008;7:123–132.

Rajasekar and Anuradha. "L-carnitine inhibits protein glycation *in vitro* and *in vivo*: evidence for a role in diabetic management." *Acta Diabetol* 2007;44:83–90.

Saraswat, et al. "Prevention of non-enzymic glycation of proteins by dietary agents: prospects for alleviating diabetic complications." *Br J Nutr* 2008; Nov: e-pub ahead of print.

Sebekova, et al. "Plasma levels of advanced glycation end-products in healthy, long-term vegetarians and subjects on a Western mixed diet." *Eur J Nutr* 2001;40:275–281.

Stirban, et al. "Benfotiamine prevents macro and microvascular endothelial dysfunction and oxidative stress following a meal rich in advanced glycation end-products in individuals with type 2 diabetes." *Diabetes Care* 2006;29:2064–2071.

Stirban, et al. "Skin autofluorescence increases postprandially in human subjects." *Diabtes Technol Ther* 2008;10:200–205.

Summa, et al. "Radical scavenging activity, anti–bacterial and mutagenic effects of cocoa bean Maillard reaction products with degree of roasting." *Mol Nutr Food Res* 2008;52:342–351.

Thirunavukkarasu, et al. "Fructose diet-induced skin collagen abnormalities are prevented by lipoic acid." *Exp Diab Res* 2004;5:237–244.

Thirunavukkarasu, et al. "Lipoic acid improves glucose utilization and prevents protein glycation and AGE formation." *Pharmazie* 2005;60:772–775.

Tsukahara, et al. "Comparison of age-related changes in facial wrinkles and sagging in the skin of Japanese, Chinese, and Thai women." *J Dermatol Sci* 2007;47:19–28.

Tsukahara, et al. "Comparison of age-related changes in facial wrinkles and sagging in the skin in Caucasian females and Japanese females." *J Cosmet Sci* 2004;55:373–385.

Tuohy, et al. "Metabolism of Maillard reaction products by the human gut microbiota—implications for health." *Mol Nutr Food Res* 2006;50:847–857.

Urbach. *Skin Diseases, Nutrition and Metabolism*. Grune & Stratton, New York, 1946.

Urbach and Lentz. "Carbohydrate metabolism and the skin." *Arch Dermatol Syphilol* 1945;52:301–316.

Uribarri and Tuttle. "Advanced glycation end-products and nephrotoxicity of high-protein diets." *Clin J Am Soc Nephrol* 2006;1:1293–1299.

Uribarri, et al. "Circulating glycotoxins and dietary advanced glycation end-products: two links to inflammatory response, oxidative stress, and aging." *J Gerontol* 2007;62A:427–433.

Uribarri, et al. "Diet-derived advanced glycation end-products are major contributors to the body's AGE pool and induce inflammation in healthy subjects." *Ann NY Acad Sci* 2005;1043:461–466.

Uribarri, et al. "Single oral challenge by advanced glycation end-products acutely impairs endotheilial function in diabetic and nondiabetic subjects." *Diabetes Care* 2007;30:2579–2582.

Urios, et al. "Flavonoids inhibit the formation of the cross-linking AGE pentosidine in collagen incubated with glucose, according to their structure." *Eur J Nutr* 2007;46:139–146.

Vlassara, et al. "Advanced glycation end-product homeostasis." *Ann NY Acad Sci* 2008;1126:46–52.

Wu and Yen. "Inhibitory effect of naturally occurring flavonoids on the formation of advanced glycation end-products." *J Agric Food Chem* 2005;53:3167–3173.

Yamagishi, et al. "Food-derived advanced glycation end-products (AGEs): a novel therapeutic target for various disorders." *Curr Pharm Design* 2007;13:2832–2836.

Yamaguchi, et al. "Collagen cross-linking in sun-exposed and unexposed sites of aged human skin." *J Invest Dermatol* 1991;97:938–941.

Chapter 4: Skin Digestion: The Gut-Skin Connection

Arnold. "Influence of food upon the bacterial flora of the small intestine." *Am J Public Health* 1927;17:918–921.

Arnold. "The passage of living bacteria through the wall of the intestine and the influence of diet and climate upon intestinal auto-infection." *Am J Hygiene* 1928;8:602–632.

Ayers. "Eczema—some recent contributions to its study." *Cal Western Med* 1930;32:153–157.

Baba, et al. "Effects of *Lactobacillus helveticus*-fermented milk on the differentiation of cultured normal epidermal keratinocytes." *J Dairy Sci* 2006;89:2072–2075.

Benno, et al. "Comparison of fecal microflora of elderly persons in rural and urban areas of Japan." *Appl Environ Microbiol* 1989;55(5):1100–1105.

Benton, et al. "Impact of consuming a milk drink containing a probiotic on mood and cognition." *Eur J Clin Nutr* 2007;61:355-361.

Blaut. "Relationship of prebiotics and food to intestinal microflora." *Eur J Nutr* 41:11–16.

Burgess. "Endogenous irritants as factors in eczema and in other dematoses." *Arch Derm Syphil* 1927;16:131–140.

Caffarelli, et al. "Elimination diet and intestinal permeability in atopic eczema: a preliminary study." *Clin Exp Allergy* 1993;23:28–31.

Caramia, et al. "Probiotics and the skin." *Clin Dermatol* 2008;26:4–11.

Card, et al. "Antibiotic use and the development of Crohn's disease." *Gut* 2004;53(2):246–250.

Chapple. "Chronic intestinal stasis treated by short-circuiting or colectomy." *Br Med J* 1911;1:915–922.

Collado, et al. "Distinct composition of gut microbiota during pregnancy in overweight and normal-weight women." *Am J Clin Nutr* 2008;88:894–899.

Di Marzio, et al. "Increase of skin-ceramide levels in aged subjects following a short-term topical application of bacterial sphingomyelinase from *Streptococcus thermophilus*." *Int J Immunopathol Pharmacol* 2008;21:137–143.

Dunlop, et al. "Abnormal intestinal permeability in subgroups of diarrhea-predominant irritable bowel syndromes." *Am J Gastroenterol* 2006;101:1288–1294.

Garrod. "Present position of the chemotherapy of bacterial infection." *Br Med J* 1955;2:756–758.

Gecse, et al. "Increased faecal serine protease activity in diarrhoeic IBS patients: a colonic luminal factor impairing colonic permeability and sensitivity." *Gut* 2008;57:591–598.

Gluck, et al. "Ingested probiotics reduce nasal colonization with pathogenic bacteria (*Staphylococcus aureus*, *Streptococcus pneumoniae*, and beta-hemolytic streptococci)." *Am J Clin Nutr* 2003;77(2):517–520.

Gordon, et al. "A *Lactobacillus* preparation for use with antibiotics." *Lancet* 1957;272:899–901.

Hara. "Influence of tea catechins on the digestive tract." *J Cell Biochem Suppl* 1997;27:52–58.

Hekmatdoost, et al. "The effect of dietary oils on cecal microflora in experimental colitis in mice." *Indian J Gastroenterol* 2008;27:186–189.

Herschell. "The therapeutical value of lactic-acid bacillus." *Proc Roy Soc Med* 1910;3:51–56.

Herter and Kendall. "The influence of dietary alternations on the types of intestinal flora." *J Biol Chem* 1909;1:203–236.

Humbert, et al. "Intestinal permeability in patients with psoriasis." *J Dermatol Sci* 1991;2:324–326.

Ivanov, et al. "Radioprotectors of the skin." *Med Radiol* 1978;23:49–58.

Jackson, et al. "Intestinal permeability in patients with eczema and food allergy." *Lancet* 1981;1:1285–1286.

Kankaanpaa, et al. "Effects of polyunsaturated fatty acids in growth medium on lipid composition and on physicochemical surface properties of *Lactobacilli*." *Appl Environ Microbiol* 2004;70(1):129–136.

Kankaanpaa, et al. "Influence of probiotic-supplemented infant formula on composition of plasma lipids in atopic infants." *J Nutr Biochem* 2002; 13(6):364–369.

Khalif, et al. "Alterations in the colonic flora and intestinal permeability and evidence of immune activation in chronic constipation." *Dig Liver Dis* 2005; 37(11):838–849.

Kirpich, et al. "Probiotics restore bowel flora and improve liver enzymes in human alcohol-induced liver injury: a pilot study." *Alcohol* 2008;42:675–682.

Koebnick, et al. "Probiotic beverage containing *Lactobacillus casei* Shirota improves gastrointestinal symptoms in patients with chronic constipation." *Can J Gastroenterol* 2003;17(11):655–659.

Kuda, et al. "Cecal environment and TBARS level in mice fed corn oil, beef tallow, and menhaden fish oil." *J Nutr Sci Vitaminol* (Tokyo) 2000 Apr;46(2):65–70.

Lane. "Chronic intestinal stasis." *Br Med J* 1913;2:1125–1128.

Maes. "Inflammatory and oxidative and nitrosative stress pathways underpinning chronic fatigue, somatization, and psychosomatic symptoms." *Curr Opin Psychiatry* 2008;22:75–83.

Maes, et al. "Normalization of the increased translocation of endotoxin from gram negative enterobacteria (leaky gut) is accompanied by a remission of chronic fatigue syndrome." *Neuroendocrinol Lett* 2007;28:739–744.

Marchetti, et al. "Efficacy of regulators of the intestinal bacterial flora in the therapy of acne vulgaris." *Clin Ter* 1987 Sep 15;122(5):339–343.

Maxwell, et al. "Antibiotics increase functional abdominal symptoms." *Am J Gastroenterol* 2002;97(1):104–108.

McCarthy, et al. "Effect of spray-dried yogurt and lactic acid bacteria on the initiation and promotion stages of chemically induced skin carcinogenesis in mice." *Nutr Cancer* 1997;27:231–237.

McNulty, et al. "The public's attitudes to and compliance with antibiotics." *J Antimicrob Chemother* 2007;60:i63–i68.

Montrose and Floch. "Probiotics used in human studies." *J Clin Gastroenterol* 2005 Jul;39(6):469–484.

Naruszewicz, et al. "Effect of *Lactobacillus plantarum* 299v on cardiovascular disease risk factors in smokers." *Am J Clin Nutr* 2002 Dec;76(6):1249–1255.

Noverr, et al. "Role of antibiotics and fungal microbiota in driving pulmonary allergic responses." *Infect Immun* 2004;72(9):4996–5003.

Nunez, et al. "Effects of psychological stress and alprazolam on development of oral candidiasis in rats." *Clin Diagn Lab Immunol* 2002 Jul;9(4):852–857.

Oh, et al. "Effect of bacteriocin produced by *Lactococcus* sp. HY 449 on skin-inflammatory bacteria." *Food Chem Toxicol* 2006;44:1184–1190.

Oxman, et al. "Oral administration of *Lactobacillus* induces cardioprotection." *J Altern Complement Med* 2001 Aug;7(4):345–354.

Peguet-Navarro, et al. "Supplementation with oral probiotic bacteria protects human cutaneous immune homeostasis after UV exposure—double-blind, randomized, placebo-controlled trial." *Eur J Dermatol* 2008;18:504–511.

Person and Bernhard. "Autointoxication revisited." *J Am Acad Derm* 1986;15:559–563.

Peyri. "Topical bacteriotherapy." *J Cutan Dis Syphil* 1912;35:1803.

Probert and Gibson. "Bacterial biofilms in the human gastrointestinal tract." *Curr Issues Intest Microbiol* 2002;3:23–27.

Puch, et al. "Consumption of functional fermented milk containing borage oil, green tea, and vitamin E enhances skin-barrier function." *Exp Dermatol* 2008;17:668–674.

Rao, et al. "A randomized, double-blind, placebo-controlled pilot study of a probiotic in emotional symptoms of chronic fatigue syndrome." *Gut Pathogens* 2009;1:6.

Rettger and Cheplin. "*Bacillus acidophilus* and its therapeutic application." *Arch Intern Med* 1922;29:357–367.

Rosell. "Yoghurt and kefir in their relation to health and therapeutics." *Can Med Assoc J* 1932;26:341–345.

Sanders. "Use of probiotics and yogurts in maintenance of health." *J Clin Gastroenterol* 2008;42:S71–S74.

Schmid-Ott. "Clinical results with a *Lactobacillus bifidus* food preparation in the treatment of skin diseases with dysbacteria." *Z Haut Geschlechtskr* 1961;30:199–203.

Scholtz. "Dermatologic therapeutics—basic principles and technique." *Cal Western Med;*33:769–774.

Shortt. "The probiotic century: historical and current perspectives." *Trends Foods Sci Technol* 1999;10:411–417.

Siver. "*Lactobacillus* for the control of acne." *J Med Soc New Jersey* 1961;59(2):52–53.

Songisepp, et al. "Evaluation of the functional efficacy of an antioxidative probiotic in healthy volunteers." *Nutr J* 2005 Aug 4;4:22.

Ten Bruggencate, et al. "Dietary fructooligosaccharides affect intestinal barrier function in healthy men." *J Nutr* 2006;136(1):70–74.

Ten Bruggencate, et al. "Dietary fructooligosaccharides increase intestinal permeability in rats." *J Nutr* 2005;135(4):837–842.

Velicer, et al. "Antibiotic use in relation to the risk of breast cancer." *JAMA*. 2004 Feb 18;291(7):827–835.

Volkova, et al. "Impact of the impaired intestinal microflora on the course of acne vulgaris." *Klin Med (Mosk)* 2001;79(6):39–41.

Walrand, et al. "Consumption of a functional fermented milk containing collagen hydrolysate improves the concentration of collagen-specific amino acids in plasma." *J Agric Food Chem* 2008;56:7790–7795.

Wang and Wu. "Effects of psychological stress on small intestinal motility and bacteria and mucosa in mice." *World J Gastroenterol* 2005 Apr 7;11(13):2016–2021.

Woodmansey. "Intestinal bacteria and ageing." *J Appl Microbiol* 2007;102:1178–1186.

Chapter 5: The Brain-Skin Connection and Your Beauty Sleep

Adam and Oswald. "Sleep helps healing." *Br Med J* 1984;289:1400–1401.

Addolorato, et al. "State and trait anxiety and depression in patients affected by gastrointestinal disease." *Int J Clin Pract* 2008;62:1063–1069.

Altemus, et al. "Stress-induced changes in skin-barrier function in healthy women." *J Invest Dermatol* 2001;117:309–317.

Arndt, et al. "Stress and atopic dermatitis." *Curr Allergy Asthma Rep* 2008;8:312–317.

Basta, et al. "Chronic insomnia and stress system." *Sleep Med Clin* 2007;2:279–291.

Bavetta, et al. "Effect of bioflavonoids and methylprednisolone on collagen biosynthesis." *Am J Physiol* 1964;206:179–182.

Bazar, et al. "A new wrinkle: skin manifestations of aging may relate to autonomic dysfunction." *Med Hypothese* 2006;67:1274–1276.

Beddoe and Murphy. "Does mindfulness decrease stress and foster empathy among nursing students?" *J Nurs Educ* 2004;43(7):305–312.

Bellisle, et al. "Non-food-related environmental stimuli induce increased meal intake in healthy women: comparison of television viewing versus listening to a recorded story in laboratory settings." *Appetite* 2004 Oct;43(2):175–180.

Beltraminelli and Itin. "Skin and psyche—from the surface to the depth of the inner world." *JDDG* 2008;6:8–14.

Benson. "Are you working too hard? A conversation with mind-body researcher Herbert Benson." *Harv Bus Rev* 2005;83(11):53–58,165.

Biro, et al. "Clinical implications of thermal therapy in lifestyle-related diseases." *Exp Biol Med* (Maywood). 2003 Nov;228(10):1245–1249.

Black, et al. "Exercise prevents age-related decline in nitric-oxide-mediated vasodilator function in cutaneous microvessels." *J Physiol* 2008;586:3511–3524.

Brown and Ryan. "The benefits of being present: mindfulness and its role in psychological well-being." *J Pers Soc Psychol* 2003;84(4):822–848.

Bulbena, et al. "Panic anxiety, under the weather?" *Int J Biometeorol* 2005 Mar;49(4):238–243.

Chesley. "Blurring boundaries? Linking technology use, spillover, individual distress, and family satisfaction." *J Marriage Fam* 2005;67:1237–1248.

Choi, et al. "Mechanisms by which psychologic stress alters cutaneous permeability barrier homeostasis and stratum corneum integrity." *J Invest Dermatol* 2005;124:587–595.

Cole-King, et al. "Psychological factors and delayed wound healing in chronic wounds." *Psychosom Med* 2001;63:216–220.

Costa, et al. "Tryptophan metabolism in animals with dermatitis." *Boll Soc Ital Biol Sper* 1979;55:1714–1720.

Darvin, et al. "One-year study on the variation of carotenoid antioxidant substances in living human skin: influence of dietary supplementation and stress factors." *J Biomed Optics* 2008;13:044028.

Davidson, et al. "Alterations in brain and immune function produced by mindfulness meditation." *Psychosom Med* 2003 Jul–Aug;65(4):564–570.

Dusek, et al. "Genomic counter-stress changes induced by the relaxation response." *PLoS One* 2008;3:e2576.

Ebercht, et al. "Perceived stress and cortisol levels predict speed of wound healing in healthy male adults." *Psychoneuroendocrinol* 2004;29:798–809.

Epel, et al. "Accelerated telomere shortening in response to life stress." *PNAS* 2004;101:17312–17315.

Esler, et al. "Chronic mental stress is a cause of essential hypertension: presence of biological markers of stress." *Clin Exp Pharmacol Physiol* 2008;35:498–502.

Esrefoglu, et al. "Ultrastructural clues for the potent therapeutic effect of melatonin on aging skin in pinealectomized rats." *Fund Clin Pharmacol* 2006;20:605–611.

Everson and Toth. "Systemic bacterial invasion induced by sleep deprivation." *Am J Physiol Regul Integr Comp Physiol* 2000;278:R905–R916.

Fields. "Call me sleepless: using a mobile phone just before bed may cause insomnia." *Sci Am Mind* 2008 Aug–Sep:6.

Fischer, et al. "Melatonin in dermatology. Experimental and clinical aspects." *Hautarzt* 1999;50:5–11.

Fors, et al. "The effect of guided imagery and amitriptyline on daily fibromyalgia pain: a prospective, randomized, controlled trial." *J Psychiatr Res* 2002;36(3):179–187.

Fox. "The influence of physical activity on mental well-being." *Public Health Nutr* 1999 Sep;2(3A):411–418.

Galvin, et al. "The relaxation response: reducing stress and improving cognition in healthy aging adults." *Complement Ther Clin Pract* 2006 Aug;12(3):186–191.

Garg, et al. "Psychological stress perturbs epidermal permeability barrier homeostasis." *Arch Dermatol* 2001;137:53–59.

Goel, et al. "Controlled trial of bright light and negative air ions for chronic depression." *Psychol Med* 2005;35(7):945–955.

Goon, et al. "Effect of tai chi exercise on DNA damage, antioxidant enzymes, and oxidative stress in middle-aged adults." *J Physical Act Health* 2009;6:43–54.

Gore, et al. "Television viewing and snacking." *Eat Behav* 2003 Nov; 4(4):399–405.

Gortner, et al. "Benefits of expressive writing in lowering rumination and depressive symptoms." *Behav Ther* 2006 Sep;37(3):292–303.

Gouin, et al. "The influence of anger expression on wound healing." *Brain Behav Immun* 2008;22:699–708.

Grebner, et al. "Working conditions and three types of well-being: a longitudinal study with self-report and rating data." *J Occup Health Psychol* 2005 Jan;10(1):31–43.

Gumustekin, et al. "Effects of sleep deprivation, nicotine, and selenium on wound healing in rats." *Int J Neurosci* 2004;114:1433–1442.

Hamer and Steptoe. "Prospective study of physical fitness, adiposity, and inflammatory markers in healthy middle-aged men and women." *Am J Clin Nutr* 2009;89:85–89.

Hill, et al. "The heart-mind connection." *Behav Healthc* 2006;26(9):30–32.

Inoue, et al. "Autonomic nervous responses according to preference for the odor of jasmine tea." *Biosci Biotechnol Biochem* 2003;67(6): 1206–1214.

Ito, et al. "GABA-synthesizing enzyme, GAD67, from dermal fibroblasts: evidence for a new skin function." *Biochimica Biophysica Acta* 2007;1770:291–296.

Iwama. "Negative air ions created by water shearing improve erythrocyte deformability and aerobic metabolism." *Indoor Air* 2004 Aug;14(4):293–297.

Jain, et al. "Effects of perceived stress and uplifts on inflammation and coagulability." *Psychophysiol* 2007;44:154–160.

Joshi. "Nonpharmacologic therapy for insomnia in the elderly." *Clin Geriatr Med* 2008;24:107–119.

Kabat-Zinn, et al. "Influence of a mindfulness meditation-based stress-reduction intervention on rates of skin clearing in patients with moderate to severe psoriasis under phototherapy (UVB) and photochemotherapy (PUVA)." *Psychosom Med* 1998;60:625–632.

Karlamangla, et al. "Reduction in allostaic load in older adults is associated with lower all-cause mortality risk: MacArthur studies of successful aging." *Psychosom Med* 2006;68:500–507.

Knowles, et al. "Investigating the role of perceived stress on bacterial flora activity and salivary cortisol secretion." *Biol Psychiatry* 2008;77:132–137.

Koh, et al. "Counter-stress effects of relaxation on proinflammatory and anti-inflammatory cytokines." *Brain Behav Immun* 2008;22:1130–1137.

Kuo and Taylor. "A potential natural treatment for attention-deficit/hyperactivity disorder: evidence from a national study." *Am J Public Health* 2004;94(9):1580–1586.

Lai and Good. "Music improves sleep quality in older adults." *J Adv Nurs* 2005 Feb;49(3):234–244.

Lee. "The effect of lavender aromatherapy on cognitive function, emotion, and aggressive behavior of elderly with dementia." *Taehan Kanho Hakhoe Chi* 2005 Apr;35(2):303–312.

Lee and Lee. "Effects of lavender aromatherapy on insomnia and depression in women college students." *Taehan Kanho Hakhoe Chi* 2006 Feb;36(1):136–143.

Leichsenring, et al. "Cognitive-behavioral therapy and psychodynamic psychotherapy: techniques, efficacy, and indications." *Am J Psychother* 2006;60(3):233–259.

Leitner, et al. "Do the effects of job stressors on health persist over time? A longitudinal study with observational stressor measures." *J Occup Health Psychol* 2005;10(1):18–30.

Lerchi, et al. "Effects of mobile phone electromagnetic fields at nonthermal SAR values on melatonin and body weight of Djungarian hamsters." *J Pineal Res* 2008;44:267–272.

Leuchter, et al. "Changes in brain function of depressed subjects during treatment with placebo." *Am J Psychiatry* 2002;159(1):122–129.

Lucas, et al. "Ethyl-eicosapentaenoic acid for the treatment of psychological distress and depressive symptoms in middle-aged women: a double-blind, placebo-controlled, randomized clinical trial." *Am J Clin Nutr* 2009;89(2):641–651.

Lutgendorf, et al. "Biobehavioral influences on matrix metalloproteinase expression in ovarian carcinoma." *Clin Cancer Res* 2008;14:6839–6846.

Manger and Motta. "The impact of an exercise program on posttraumatic stress disorder, anxiety, and depression." *Int J Emerg Ment Health* 2005 Winter;7(1):49–57.

Masuda, et al. "The effects of repeated thermal therapy for patients with chronic pain." *Psychother Psychosom* 2005;74(5):288–294.

Masuda, et al. "Repeated sauna therapy reduces urinary 8-epi-prostaglandin F(2alpha)." *Jpn Heart J* 2004 Mar;45(2):297–303.

McCraty, et al. "The effects of different types of music on mood, tension, and mental clarity." *Altern Ther Health Med* 1998;4(1):75–84.

McDade, et al. "Psychosocial and behavioral predictors of inflammation in middle-aged and older adults: the Chicago health, aging, and social relations study." *Psychosom Med* 2006;68:376–381.

Michalsen, et al. "Rapid stress reduction and anxiolysis among distressed women as a consequence of a three-month intensive yoga program." *Med Sci Monit* 2005;11(12):CR555–561.

Miura, et al. "A link between stress and depression: shifts in the balance between the kynurenine and serotonin pathways of tryptophan metabolism and the etiology and pathophysiology of depression." *Stress* 2008;11:198–209.

Morimoto, et al. "Possible involvement of prostaglandins in psychological stress-induced responses in rats." *J Physiol* 1991;443:421–429.

Morita, et al. "Psychological effects of forest environments on healthy adults: *shinrin-yoku* (forest-air bathing, walking) as a possible method of stress reduction." *Public Health* 2007;121(1):54–63.

Moss, et al. "Aromas of rosemary and lavender essential oils differentially affect cognition and mood in healthy adults." *Int J Neurosci* 2003;113(1):15–38.

Mullington, et al. "Cardiovascular, inflammatory, and metabolic consequences of sleep deprivation." *Progress Cardiovasc Dis* 2009;51: 294–302.

Nakane, et al. "Effect of negative air ions on computer operation, anxiety, and salivary chromogranin A-like immunoreactivity." *Int J Psychophysiol* 2002 Oct;46(1):85–89.

Nedeltcheva, et al. "Sleep curtailment is accompanied by increased intake of calories from snacks." *Am J Clin Nutr* 2009;89:126–133.

Nijm and Jonasson. "Inflammation and cortisol response in coronary artery disease." *Ann Med* 2009;41(3):224–233.

Nordlind, et al. "The skin as a mirror of the soul: exploring the possible roles of serotonin." *Exp Dermatol* 2007;17:301–311.

Norrish and Dwyer. "Preliminary investigation of the effect of peppermint oil on an objective measure of daytime sleepiness." *Int J Psychophysiol* 2005;55(3):291–298.

Ohtsuka, et al. "*Shinrin-yoku* (forest-air bathing and walking) effectively decreases blood glucose levels in diabetic patients." *Int J Biometeorol* 1998 Feb;41(3):125–127.

Oikarinen, et al. "The molecular basis of glucocorticoid-induced skin atrophy: topical glucocorticoid apparently decreases both collagen synthesis and the corresponding collagen mRNA level in human skin *in vivo*." *Br J Dermatol* 1998;139:1106–1110.

Ono, et al. "A pilot study of the relationship between bowel habits and sleep health by actigraphy measurement and fecal flora analysis." *J Physiol Anthropol* 2008;27:145–151.

Ornish, et al. "Increased telomerase activity and comprehensive lifestyle changes: a pilot study." *Lancet Oncol* 2008;9:1048–1057.

Pardon. "Stress and ageing interactions: a paradox in the context of shared etiological and physiopathological processes." *Brain Res Rev* 2007;54:251–273.

Park, et al. "Physiological effects of *shinrin-yoku* (taking in the atmosphere of the forest)—using salivary cortisol and cerebral activity as indicators." *J Physiol Anthropol* 2007 Mar;26(2):123–128.

Pennebaker. "The effects of traumatic disclosure on physical and mental health: the values of writing and talking about upsetting events." *Int J Emerg Ment Health* 1999 Winter;1(1):9–18.

Pergams and Zaradic. "Evidence for a fundamental and pervasive shift away from nature-based recreation." *PNAS* 2008;105:2295–2300.

Riemann, et al. "The tryptophan depletion test: impact on sleep in primary insomnia—a pilot study." *Psychiatr Res* 2002;109:129–135.

Robles. "Stress, social support, and delayed skin barrier recovery." *Psychosom Med* 2007;69:807–815.

Saeki, et al. "The effect of footbath with or without the essential oil of lavender on the autonomic nervous system: a randomized trial." *Complement Ther Med* 2000 Mar;8(1):2–7.

Saul. "Psycho-physiological stress and its effect on ultraviolet light-induced inflammation, DNA damage, and skin carcinogenesis." *Rejuv Res* 2007;10:642.

Schulz, et al. "Increased free cortisol secretion after awakening in chronically stressed individuals due to work overload." *Stress Med* 1998;14:91–97.

Scutt, et al. "Stimulation of human fibroblast collagen synthesis *in vitro* by gamma-aminobutyric acid." *Biochem Pharmacol* 1987;36:1333–1335.

Shenefelt. "Therapeutic management of psychodermatological disorders." *Expert Opin Pharmacother* 2008;9:973–985.

Slominski. "A nervous breakdown in the skin: stress and the epidermal barrier." *J Clin Invest* 2007;117:3166–169.

Solberg, et al. "The effects of long meditation on plasma melatonin and blood serotonin." *Med Sci Monit* 2004;10(3):CR96–101.

Steptoe, et al. "Job strain and anger expression predict early-morning elevations in salivary cortisol." *Psychosom Med* 2000;62:286–292.

Stokes and Pillsbury. "The effect on the skin of emotional and nervous states." *Arch Dermatol Syphilol* 1930;22:962–993.

Streeter, et al. "Yoga asana sessions increase brain GABA levels: a pilot study." *J Altern Complem Med* 2007;13:419–426.

Strohle, et al. "The acute antipanic activity of aerobic exercise." *Am J Psychiatry* 2005;162(12):2376–2378.

Suess, et al. "The effects of psychological stress on respiration: a preliminary study of anxiety and hyperventilation." *Psychophysiol* 1980;17:535–540.

Sugimoto, et al. "Telomere length of the skin in association with chronological aging and photoaging." *J Dermatol Sci* 2006;43:43–47.

Sundquist, et al. "Urbanisation and incidence of psychosis and depression: follow-up study of 4.4 million women and men in Sweden." *Br J Psychiatry* 2004 Apr;184:293–298.

Tanida, et al. "Effects of fragrance administration on stress-induced prefrontal cortex activity and sebum secretion in the facial skin." *Neurosci Lett* 2008;432:157–161.

Tazawa and Okada. "Physical signs associated with excessive television-game playing and sleep deprivation." *Pediatr Int* 2001;43:647–650.

Tsunetsugu, et al. "Physiological effects of *shinrin-yoku* (taking in the atmosphere of the forest) in an old-growth broadleaf forest in Yamagata Prefecture, Japan." *J Physiol Anthropol* 2007 Mar;26(2):135–142.

Uhe, et al. "A comparison of the effects of beef, chicken, and fish protein on satiety and amino acid profiles in lean healthy subjects." *J Nutr* 1992;122:467–472.

Varga, et al. "Control of extracellular matrix degradation by interferon gamma. The tyrptophan connection." *Adv Exp Med Biol* 1996;398:143–148.

Vasquez, et al. "Associations of dietary intake and physical activity with sleep-disordered breathing in the Apnea Positive Pressure Long-Term Efficacy Study (APPLES)." *J Clin Sleep Med* 2008 Oct 15;4(5):411–418.

Vitetta, et al. "Mind-body medicine." *Ann NY Acad Sci* 2005;1057:492–505.

Watanabe, et al. "Differences in relaxation by means of guided imagery in a healthy community sample." *Altern Ther Health Med* 2006;12(2):60–66.

West, et al. "Effects of Hatha yoga and African dance on perceived stress, affect, and salivary cortisol." *Ann Behav Med* 2004 Oct;28(2):114–118.

Wilkinson and Barczak. "Psychiatric screening in general practice: comparison of the general health questionnaire and the hospital anxiety depression scale." *J Roy Coll Gen Pract* 1988;38:311–313.

Winkelman, et al. "Reduced brain GABA in primary insomnia." *Sleep* 2008;31:1499–1506.

Yamaguchi, et al. "The effects of exercise in forest and urban environments on sympathetic nervous activity of normal young adults." *J Int Med Res.* 2006;34(2):152–159.

Yook, et al. "Usefulness of mindfulness-based cognitive therapy for treating insomnia in patients with anxiety disorders." *J Nerv Ment Dis* 2008;196:501–503.

Zoumakis, et al. "The 'brain-skin connection': nerve growth factor–dependent pathways for stress-induced skin disorders." *J Mol Med* 2007;85:1347–1349.

Chapter 6: Skin Food I: Dietary Supplements

Abdel-Kader, et al. "Stabilization of mitochondrial function by *Ginkgo biloba* extract (EGB 761)." *Pharmacol Res* 2007;56:493–502.

Abidov, et al. "Effect of extracts from *Rhodiola rosea* and *Rhodiola crenulata* roots on ATP content in mitochondria of skeletal muscles." *Bull Exp Biol Med* 2003;136:585–587.

Ames. "A role for supplements in optimizing health: the metabolic tune-up." *Arch Biochem Biophys* 2004;423:227–234.

Ames, et al. "Mineral and vitamin deficiencies can accelerate the mitochondrial decay of aging." *Mol Aspects Med* 2005;26:363–378.

Anderson. "Foods as the cause of acne." *Am Fam Physician* 1971;3(3): 102–103.

Ashida, et al. "CoQ_{10} supplementation elevates the epidermal CoQ_{10} level in adult hairless mice." *Biofactors* 2005;25:175–178.

Ashida, et al. "Effect of Co-enzyme Q_{10} as a supplement on wrinkle reduction." *Food Style* 2004;6:1–4.

Balogh, et al. "Absorption, uptake, and tissue affinity of high-molecular-weight hyaluronan after oral administration in rats and dogs." *J Agric Food Chem.* 2008;56:10582–93.

Barel, et al. "Effect of oral intake of choline-stabilized orthosilicic acid on skin, nails, and hair in women with photodamaged skin." *Arch Dermatol Res* 2005;297:147–153.

Berardi, et al. "Plant-based dietary supplement increases urinary pH." *J Int Soc Sports Nutr* 2008;5:20.

Brosche and Platt. "Effect of borage-oil consumption on fatty acid metabolism, transepidermal water loss, and skin parameters in elderly people." *Arch Gerontol Geriatr* 2000;30:139–150.

Davis, et al. "Quercetin increases brain and muscle mitochondrial biogenesis and exercise tolerance." *Am J Physiol Regul Integr Comp Physiol* 2009;296:R1071–R1077.

De Spirt, et al. "Intervention with flaxseed and borage-oil supplements modulates skin condition in women." *Br J Nutr* 2008;101:440–445.

Distante, et al. "Oral fish cartilage polysaccharides in the treatment of photoageing: biophysical findings." *Int J Cosmet Sci* 2002;24:81–87.

Elias. "Does the tail wag the dog? Role of the barrier in the pathogenesis of inflammatory dermatoses." *Arch Dermatol* 2001;137:1079–1081.

Eskelinin and Santalahti. "Special natural cartilage polysaccharides for the treatment of sun-damaged skin in females." *J Int Med Res* 1992;20:99–105.

Gueniche, et al. "*Lactobacillus johnsonii* provides a dose-dependent protection against UVR-induced immunosuppression." *Eur J Dermatol* 2008;18:476–477.

Heinrich, et al. "Supplementation with nutritional cartilage extract positively influences skin hydration, skin barrier, and skin structure." *Int J Cosmet Sci* 2007;29:144–145.

Heller, et al. "Top-10 list of herbal and supplemental medicines used by cosmetic patients." *Plast Reconstruct Surg* 2006;117:436–445.

Hollenberg, et al. "Is it the dark in dark chocolate?" *Circulation* 2007; 116;2360–2362.

Izumi, et al. "Oral intake of soy isoflavone aglycone improves the aged skin of adult women." *J Nutr Sci Vitaminol* 2007;53:57–62.

Jacquet, et al. "Effect of dietary supplementation with Inversion Femme on slimming, hair loss, and skin and nail parameters in women." *Adv Ther* 2007;24:1154–1171.

Jeon, et al. "Effects of oral epigallocatechin gallate supplementation on the minimal erythema dose and UV-induced skin damage." *Skin Pharmacol Physiol* 2009;22:137–141.

Jugdaohsingh, et al. "Dietary silicon intake and absorption." *Am J Clin Nutr* 2002;75:887–893.

Jugdaohsingh, et al. "Dietary silicon intake is positively associated with bone mineral density in men and premenopausal women of the Framingham Offspring Cohort." *J Bone Miner Res* 2004;19:297–307.

Kieffer and Efsen. "Imedeen in the treatment of photoaged skin: an efficacy and safety trial over 12 months." *J Eur Acad Dermatol Venereol* 1998;11:129–136.

Kimata. "Improvement of atopic dermatitis and reduction of skin allergic responses by oral intake of konjac ceramide." *Pediatr Dermatol* 2006;23:386–389.

Kurd, et al. "Oral curcumin in the treatment of moderate to severe psoriasis vulgaris." *J Am Acad Dermatol* 2008;58:625–631.

Lassus, et al. "Imedeen for the treatment of degenerated skin in females." *J Int Med Res* 1991;19:147–152.

Lubowe. "A modern approach to the treatment of aging skin." *J Appl Nutr* 1979;31:64–66.

Mac-Mary, et al. "Could a photobiological test be a suitable method to assess the antioxidant effect of a nutritional supplement (Glisodin)." *Eur J Dermatol* 2007;17:254–255.

Maurer, et al. "Neutralization of Western diet inhibits bone resorption independently of K intake and reduces cortisol secretion in humans." *Am J Physiol Renal Physiol* 2003;284:F32–40.

Messina, et al. "Estimated Asian adult soy protein and isoflavone intake." *Nutr Cancer* 2006;55:1–12.

Minich and Bland. "Acid-alkaline balance: role in chronic disease and detoxification." *Altern Ther* 2007;13:62–65.

Miyanishi, et al. "Reduction of transepidermal water loss by oral intake of glucosylceramides in patients with atopic eczema." *Allergy* 2005;60: 1454–1455.

Moehrle, et al. "Sun protection by red wine?" *JDDG* 2009;7:29–32.

Morganti, et al. "Role of topical and nutritional supplement to modify the oxidative stress." *Int J Cosmet Sci* 2002;24:331–339.

Muggli. "Systemic evening primrose oil improves the biophysical skin parameters of healthy adults." *Int J Cosmet Sci* 2005;27:243–249.

Pei, et al. "Effect of marine collagen peptide on delaying the skin aging." *Zhonghua Yu Fang Yi Xue Za Zhi* 2008;42:235–238.

Pepe. "Effect of dietary polyunsaturated fatty acids on age-related changes in cardiac mitochondrial membranes." *Exp Gerontol* 2005;40:751–758.

Primavera and Berardesca. "Clinical and instrumental evaluation of a food supplement in improving skin hydration." *Int J Cosmet Sci* 2005;27:199–204.

Puch, et al. "Consumption of functional fermented milk containing borage oil, green tea, and vitamin E enhances skin-barrier function." *Exp Dermatol* 2008;17(8):668–674.

Regnault, et al. "Pharmacokinetics of superoxide dismutase in rats after oral administration." *Biopharm Drug Disposition* 1996;17:165–174.

Rona and Berardesca. "Aging skin and food supplements: the myth and the truth." *Clin Dermatol* 2008;26:641–647.

Segger and Schonlau. "Supplementation with Evelle improves skin smoothness and elasticity in a double-blind, placebo-controlled study with 62 women." *J Dermatol Treatment* 2004;15:222–226.

Segger, et al. "Supplementation with Eskimo Skin Care improves skin elasticity in women." *J Dermatol Treat* 2008;19:279–283.

Sharma, et al. "Dietary grape seed proanthocyanidins inhibit UVB-induced oxidative stress and activation of mitogen-activated protein kinases and nuclear factor-κ B signaling in *in vivo* SKH-1 hairless mice." *Mol Cancer The* 2007;6:995–1005.

Sinclair. "The vitamin B complex." *Postgrad Med J* 1941;17:3–12.

Skovgaard, et al. "Effect of a novel dietary supplement on skin aging in post-menopausal women." *Eur J Clin Nutr* 2006;60:1201–1206.

Stahl, et al. "Lycopene-rich products and dietary photoprotection." *Photochem Photobiol Sci* 2006;5:238–242.

Steenvoorden, et al. "The use of endogenous antioxidants to improve photoprotection." *J Photochem Photobiol* 1997;41:1–10.

Stokes, et al. "Carbohydrate and water metabolism and the vitamins in skin inflammation." *Am J Med Sci* 1938;195:562–574.

Sumida, et al. "The effect of oral ingestion of collagen peptide on skin hydration and biochemical data of blood." *J Nutr Food* 2004;7:45–52.

Takemura, et al. "Dietary, but not topical, alpha-linolenic acid suppresses UVB-induced skin injury in hairless mice when compared with linoleic acid." *Photochem Photobiol* 2002;76:657–663.

Thom. "A randomized, double-blind, placebo-controlled study on the clinical efficacy of oral treatment with Dermavite on aging symptoms of the skin." *J Int Med Res* 2005;33:267–272.

Tsuji, et al. "Dietary glucosylceramide improves skin-barrier function in hairless mice." *J Dermatol Sci* 2006;44:101–107.

Walrand, et al. "Consumption of a functional fermented milk containing collagen hydrolysate improves the concentration of collagen-specific amino acids in plasma." *J Agric Food Chem* 2008;56:7790–7795.

Yiasemides, et al. "Oral nicotinamide protects against ultraviolet radiation-induced immunosuppression in humans." *Carcinogenesis* 2009;30:101–105.

Zague. "A new view concerning the effects of collagen hydrolysate intake on skin properties." *Arch Dermatol Res* 2008;300:479–483.

Chapter 7: Skin Food II: Natural Topicals and Concluding Remarks

Ahshawat, et al. "Preparation and characterization of herbal creams for improvement of skin viscoelastic properties." *Int J Cosmet Sci* 2008;30:183–193.

Andreassi, et al. "Antioxidant activity of topically applied lycopene." *Eur J Dermatol Venereol* 2004;18:52–55.

Baumann. "Botanical ingredients in cosmeceuticals." *J Drugs Dermatol* 2007;6:1084–1088.

Baumann. "Less known botanical cosmeceuticals." *Dermatol Ther* 2007;20:330–342.

Baxter. "Anti-aging properties of resveratrol: review and report of a potent new antioxidant skin care formulation." *J Cosmet Dermatol* 2008;7:2–7.

Behrman, et al. "Dermatologic therapy with cod-liver oil ointment." *Ind Med Surg* 1949;18:512–518.

Beitner, et al. "Randomized, placebo-controlled, double-blind study on the clinical efficacy of a cream containing 5 percent alpha-lipoic acid related to photoageing of facial skin." *Br J Dermatol* 2003;149:841–849.

Berardesca, et al. "Combined effects of silymarin and MSM in the management of rosacea." *J Cosmet Sci* 2008;7:8–14.

Bissett, et al. "Topical niacinamide reduces yellowing, wrinkling, red blotchiness, and hyperpigmented spots in aging facial skin." *Int J Cosmet Sci* 2004;26:231–238.

Blatt, et al. "Stimulation of skin's energy metabolism provides multiple benefits for mature human skin." *Biofactors* 2005;25:179–185.

Bonina, et al. "*In vitro* antioxidant activity and *in vivo* photoprotective effect of a red orange extract." *Int J Cosmet Sci* 1998;20:331–342.

Bruce. "Complementary effects of topical antiaging treatments in conjunction with aesthetic procedures." *J Drugs Dermatol* 2008;7:S23–S27.

Burgess. "Topical vitamins." *J Drugs Dermatol* 2008;7:S2–S6.

Casagrande, et al. "Protective effect of topical formulations containing quercetin against UVB-induced oxidative stress in hairless mice." *J Photochem Photobiol* 2006;84:21–27.

Chen, et al. "Nondenatured soy extracts reduce UVB-induced skin damage via multiple mechanisms." *Photochem Photobiol* 2008;84:1551–1559.

Cho, et al. "Phosphatidylserine prevents UV-induced decrease of type I procollagen and increase of MMP-1 in dermal fibroblasts and human skin *in vivo.*" *J Lipid Res* 2009;49:1235–1245.

Damian, et al. "UV radiation–induced immunosuppression is greater in men and prevented by topical nicotinamide." *J Invest Dermatol* 2008;128:447–454.

Darvin, et al. "Effect of supplemented and topically applied antioxidant substances on human tissue." *Skin Pharmacol Physiol* 2006;19:238–247.

Di Mambro and Fonseca. "Assessment of physical and antioxidant activity stability, *in vitro* release and *in vivo* efficacy of formulations added with superoxide dismutase alone or in association with alpha-tocopherol." *Eur J Pham Biopharm* 2007;66:451–459.

Di Marzio, et al. "Effect of lactic acid bacterium *Streptococcus thermophilus* on stratum corneum ceramide levels and signs and symptoms of atopic dermatitis patients." *Exp Dermatol* 2003;12:615–620.

Di Marzio, et al. "Increase of skin-ceramide levels in aged subjects following a short-term topical application of bacterial sphingomyelinase from *Streptococcus thermophilis.*" *Int J Immunopathol Pharmacol* 2008;21:137–143.

Dieamant, et al. "Neuroimmunomodulatory compound for sensitive skin care: *in vitro* and clinical assessment." *J Cosmet Dermatol* 2008;7: 112–119.

Dinkova-Kostova, et al. "Induction of the phase 2 response in mouse and human skin by sulforaphane-containing broccoli sprout extracts." *Cancer Epidemiol Biomarkers Prev* 2007;16:847–851.

Fiorani, et al. "Mitochondria accumulate large amounts of quercetin." *J Nutr Biochem* 2009;Mar 17:e-pub ahead of print.

Fujimura, et al. "A horse chestnut extract, which induces contraction forces in fibroblasts, is a potent anti-aging ingredient." *Int J Cosme Sci* 2007;29:140.

Gasser, et al. "Cocoa polyphenols and their influence on parameters involved in *ex vivo* skin restructuring." *Int J Cosmet Sci* 2008;30:339–345.

Grether-Beck, et al. "Topical application of vitamins, phyosterols, and ceramides. Protection against increased expression of interstitial collagenase and reduced collagen-1 expression after single exposure to UVA radiation." *Hautarzt* 2008;59:557–562.

Gupta and Gilchrest. "Psychosocial aspects of aging skin." *Dermatol Clin* 2005;23:643–648.

Gupta and Gupta. "Dissatisfaction with skin appearance among patients with eating disorders and non-clinical controls." *Br J Dermatol* 2001;145:110–113.

Gupta, et al. "Effects of *Rhodiola imbricate* on dermal wound healing." *Planta Med* 2007;73:774–777.

Hanson, et al. "Sunscreen enhancement of UV-induced reactive oxygen species in the skin." *Free Radic Med* 2006;41:1205–1212.

Huang, et al. "Biological and pharmacological activities of squalene and related compounds: potential uses in cosmetic dermatology." *Molecules* 2009;14:540–554.

Huang, et al. "*In vitro* and *in vivo* evaluation of topical delivery and potential dermal use of soy isoflavones genistein and daidzein." *Int J Pharm* 2008;364:36–44.

Huang, et al. "Transport of aspalathin, a rooibos tea flavonoid, across the skin and intestinal epithelium." *Phytother Res* 2008;22:699–704.

Hung, et al. "Delivery of resveratrol, a red wine polyphenol, from solutions and hydrogels via the skin." *Bio Pharm Bull* 2008;31:955–962.

Hwang, et al. "Photochemoprevention of UVB-induced skin carcinogenesis in SKH-1 mice by brown algae polyphenols." *Int J Cancer* 2006;119:2742–2749.

Isnard, et al. "Pharmacology of skin aging. Stimulation of glycosaminoglycan biosynthesis by L-fucose and fucose-rich polysaccharides, effect of *in vitro* aging of fibroblasts." *Biomed Pharm* 2004;58:202–204.

Jackson. "Connective tissue growth stimulated by carrageenin." *Biochem J* 1957;65:277–284.

Joo, et al. "Therapeutic advantages of medicinal herbs fermented with *Lactobacillus plantarum*, in topical application and its activities on atopic dermatitis." *Phytother Res* 2009; Jan 14: e-pub ahead of print.

Kafi, et al. "Improvement of naturally aged skin with vitamin A (retinol)." *Arch Dermatol* 2007;143:606–612.

Kanehara, et al. "Clinical effects of undershirts coated with borage oil on children with atopic dermatitis: a double-blind, placebo-controlled clinical trial." *J Dermatol* 2007;34:811–815.

Kang, et al. "Caffeic acid, a phenolic phytochemical in coffee, directly inhibits Fyn kinase activity and UVB-induced COX-2 expression." *Carcinogenesis* 2009;30(2):321–330.

Katiyar, et al. "Silymarin, a flavonoid from milk thistle, inhibits UV-induced oxidative stress through targeting infiltrating CD11b cells in mouse skin." *Photochem Photobiol* 2008;84:266–271.

Kawada, et al. "Evaluation of anti-wrinkle effects of a novel cosmetic containing niacinamide." *J Dermatol* 2008;35:637–642.

Khan, et al. "Effects of the brown seaweed *Undaria pinnatifida* on erythematous inflammation assessed using digital photo analysis." *Phytother Res* 2008;22:634–639.

Kim, et al. "6-gingerol prevents UVB-induced ROS production and COX-2 expression *in vitro* and *in vivo*." *Free Radic Res* 2007;41:603–614.

Kim, et al. "Photoprotective and anti-skin-aging effects of eicosapentaenoic acid in human skin *in vivo*." *J Lipid Res* 2006;47:921–930.

Knott, et al. "A novel treatment option for photoaged skin." *J Cosmet Dermatol* 2008;7:15–22.

Knott, et al. "Natural *Arctium lappa* fruit extract improves the clinical signs of aging skin." *J Cosmet Dermatol* 2008;7:281–289.

Kohlenzer. "Psycosocial aspects of beauty: how and why to look good." *Clin Dermatol* 2003;21:473–475.

Koya-Miyata, et al. "Identification of a collagen production-promoting factor from an extract of royal jelly and its possible mechanism." *Biosci Biotechnol Biochem* 2004;68:767–773.

Kwak, et al. "Effects of ginkgetin from *Ginkgo biloba* leaves on cyclooxygenases and *in vivo* skin inflammation." *Planta Med* 2002;68:316–321.

Lee, et al. "Evaluation of the effects of a preparation containing asiaticoside on periocular wrinkles of human volunteers." *Int J Cosmet Sci* 2008;30:167–173.

Lu, et al. "Tumorigenic effect of some commonly used moisturizing creams when applied topically to UVB-pretreated high-risk mice." *J Invest Dermatol* 2009;129:468–475.

Martin, et al. "Parthenolide-depleted feverfew protects skin from UV irradiation and external aggression." *Arch Dermatol* 2008;300:69–80.

Minghetti, et al. "Evaluation of the topical anti-inflammatory activity of ginger dry extracts from solutions and plasters." *Planta Med* 2007;73:1525–1530.

Mitani, et al. "Topical application of plant extracts containing xanthine derivatives can prevent UV-induced wrinkle formation in hairless mice." *Photoderm Photoimmunol Photomed* 2007;23:86–94.

Miyazaki, et al. "Topical application of Bifidobacterium-fermented soy milk extract containing genistein and diadzein improves rheological and physiological properties of skin." *J Cosmet Sci* 2004;55:473–479.

Molina. "Omega ceramide technology." *Household Personal Care Today* 2008;2:12–15.

Morvan and Vallee. "Effect of microalgal extracts on thioredoxin expression in human skin cells and their protection of skin." *Int J Cosmet Sci* 2008;30:76.

Murray, et al. "A topical antioxidant solution containing vitamins C and E stabilized by ferulic acid provides protection for human skin against damage caused by ultraviolet irradiation." *J Am Acad Dermatol* 2008;59:418–425.

Murthy, et al. "Study on wound healing activity of *Purnica granatum* peel." *J Med Food* 2004;7:256–259.

Nakahara, et al. "Effect of sake concentrate on the epidemis of aged mice and confirmation of ethy α-D-Glucoside as its active component." *Biosci Biotechnol Biochem* 2007;71:427–434.

Oh, et al. "Effect of bacteriocin produced by *Lactococcus* sp. HY 449 on skin-inflammatory bacteria." *Food Chem Toxicol* 2006;44:1184–1190.

Oresajo, et al. "Protective effects of a topical antioxidant mixture containing vitamin C, ferulic acid, and phloretin against ultraviolet-induced photodamage in human skin." *J Cosmet Sci* 2008;7:290–297.

Pacheco-Palencia, et al. "Protective effects of standardized pomegranate polyphenolic extract in ultraviolet-irradiated human skin fibroblasts." *J Agric Food Chem* 2008;56:8434–8441.

Pajonk, et al. "The effects of tea extracts on proinflammatory signaling." *BMC Medicine* 2006;4:28.

Patel, et al. "Formulation and evaluation of curcumin gel for topical application." *Pharm Dev Technol* 2009;14:80–89.

Patel, et al. "Polymeric black tea polyphenols inhibit mouse skin chemical carcinogenesis by decreasing cell proliferation." *Cell Prolif* 2008;41:532–553.

Peral, et al. "Bacteriotherapy with *Lactobacillus plantarum* in burns." *Int Wound J* 2009;6:73–81.

Prahl, et al. "Aging skin is functionally anaerobic: importance of Co-enzyme Q_{10} for anti–aging skin care." *Biofactors* 2008;32:245–255.

Prashar, et al. "Cytotoxicity of lavender oil and its major components to human skin cells." *Cell Prolif* 2004;37:221–229.

Puglia and Bonina. "*In vivo* spectrophotometric evaluation of skin-barrier recovery after topical application of soybean phytosterols." *J Cosmet Sci* 2008;59:217–224.

Ramos-e-Silva, et al. "Hydrox acids and retinoids in cosmetics." *Clin Dermatol* 2001;19:460–466.

Robert, et al. "Effect of a preparation containing a fucose-rich polysaccharide on periorbital wrinkles of human voluntaries." *Skin Res Technol* 2005;11:47–52.

Seo, et al. "Anti-aging effect of rice wine in cultured human fibroblasts and keratinocytes." *J Biosci Bioengineer* 2009;107:266–271.

Sharma, et al. "Development and evaluation of sesamol as an anti-aging agent." *Int J Dermatol* 2006;45:200–208.

Sommerfeld. "Randomized, placebo-controlled, double-blind, split-face study on the clinical efficacy of Tricutan on skin firmness." *Phytomed* 2007;14:711–715.

Stucker, et al. "Topical vitamin B_{12}—a new therapeutic approach in atopic dermatitis." *Br J Dermatol* 2004;150:977–983.

Talalay, et al. "Sulforaphane mobilizes cellular defenses that protect skin against damage by UV radiation." *PNAS* 2007;104:17500–17505.

Thomas and Heard. "*In vitro* transcutaneous delivery of ketoprofen and essential polyunsaturated fatty acids from a fish oil vehicle incorporating 1,8-cineole." *Drug Deliv* 2005;12:7–14.

Thorne. "Topical tretinoin research: an historical perspective." *J Int Med Res* 1990;18:18C–25C.

Tsoyi, et al. "Protective effect of anthocyanins from black soybean seed coats on UVB-induced apoptotic cell death *in vitro* and *in vivo*." *J Agric Food Chem* 2008;56:10600–10605.

Tsu, et al. "Evaluating the efficacy in improving facial photodamage with a mixture of topical antioxidants." *J Drugs Dermatol* 2007;6:1141–1148.

Tsukahara, et al. "Inhibition of ultraviolet B–induced wrinkle formation by an elastase-inhibiting herbal extract." *Int J Dermatol* 2006;45:460–468.

Tsukahara, et al. "Selective inhibition of skin fibroblast elastase elicits a concentration-dependent prevention of ultraviolet B–induced wrinkle formation." *J Invest Dermatol* 2001;117:671–677.

Unui, et al. "Mechanisms of inhibitory effects of CoQ_{10} on UVB-induced wrinkle formation *in vitro* and *in vivo*." *Biofactors* 2008;32:237–243.

Vayalil, et al. "Treatment of green tea polyphenols in hydrophilic cream prevents UVB-induced oxidation of lipids and proteins, depletion of antioxidant enzymes, and phosphorylation of MAPK proteins in SHK-1 hairless mouse skin." *Carcinogenesis* 2003;24:927–936.

Viola and Viola. "Virgin olive oil as a fundamental nutritional component and skin protector." *Clin Dermatol* 2009;27:159–165.

Wallo, et al. "Efficacy of a soy moisturizer in photoaging: a double-blind, vehicle-controlled, 12-week study." *J Drugs Dermatol* 2007;6:917–922.

Zaika, et al. "Inhibition of lactic acid bacteria by herbs." *J Food Sci* 1983;48:1455–1459.

Zemtsov. "Skin phosphocreatine." *Skin Res Technol* 2007;13:115–118.

Zulfakar, et al. "Is there a role for topically delivered eicosapentaenoic acid in the treatment of psoriasis?" *Eur J Dermatol* 2007;17:284–291.

Index

Wine, 195–196

Wireless technology. *See* Cell phones;
    Electromagnetic frequencies (EMF)

Wrinkles, 1, 12–15, 16

X

Xanax, 98

Y

Yakult, 71, 249

Yeast, 144

Yoga, 131–132

Yogurt, 42, 77, 96, 152, 171–172, 204

Z

Zeaxanthin, 51, 52, 149

Zinc, 19, 23, 122, 124, 151, 163

About the Authors

Alan C. Logan, ND FRSH, is a board-certified naturopathic physician who is licensed in Connecticut. He graduated magna cum laude from the State University of New York at Purchase and as valedictorian from the Canadian College of Naturopathic Medicine. As an invited faculty member of Harvard's School of Continuing Medical Education, Logan lectures in the mind-body medicine courses offered at Harvard. Coauthor of *The Clear Skin Diet* (Sourcebooks, 2007), he is the only naturopathic doctor to have had his commentaries published in the four leading dermatology journals—*Archives of Dermatology*, the *International Journal of Dermatology*, the *Journal of the American Academy of Dermatology*, and the *British Journal of Dermatology*. Widely regarded as one of North America's leading cosmetic nutritionists, he has been featured in health and beauty magazines such as *Cosmopolitan*, *Elle*, *W*, and *Life & Style*, as well as on *CTV* and *Global National* Canadian television.

Mark G. Rubin, MD, is a board-certified dermatologist and assistant professor of dermatology at the University of California, San Diego. In addition, he has a private practice devoted exclusively to cosmetic dermatology in Beverly Hills, California. Rubin is the author of two books and numerous articles on skin rejuvenation. He has personally trained more than six hundred physicians in his techniques for skin rejuvenation and has lectured on those techniques in more than ten countries. Over the past fifteen years, Rubin has been involved in clinical research, including several FDA trials, and he is a consultant to multiple medical device, cosmetic, and pharmaceutical companies. He also has been a resource for leading health and beauty magazines.

Phillip M. Levy, MD, is licensed in internal medicine and dermatology in the United States and Switzerland. A pioneer in cosmetic dermatology, Levy is widely recognized for having discovered a variety of skin-rejuvenating techniques. Many of the esthetic dermatology techniques that he pioneered are now widely used by cosmetic dermatologists. An assistant clinical professor of dermatology at the Université de Franche-Comté in Besançon, France, he is the author of many scientific articles and book chapters on dermatology and esthetic subjects. Currently practicing in Geneva, Switzerland, he has been featured on many European TV programs and in newspaper and magazine articles.